P9-ELV-203

CARDIOLOGY
IN FAMILY PRACTICE

CURRENT CLINICAL PRACTICE

NEIL S. SKOLNIK, MD SERIES EDITOR

Cardiology
in Family Practice

A Practical Guide

Steven M. Hollenberg, MD
Tracy Walker, MD

Cooper University Hospital,
Robert Wood Johnson Medical School,
University of Medicine and Dentistry of New Jersey
Camden, NJ

HUMANA PRESS ✱ TOTOWA, NEW JERSEY

© 2006 Humana Press Inc.
999 Riverview Drive, Suite 208
Totowa, New Jersey 07512

humanapress.com

Due diligence has been taken by the publishers, editors, and authors of this book to assure the accuracy of the information published and to describe generally accepted practices. The contributors herein have carefully checked to ensure that the drug selections and dosages set forth in this text are accurate and in accord with the standards accepted at the time of publication. Notwithstanding, as new research, changes in government regulations, and knowledge from clinical experience relating to drug therapy and drug reactions constantly occurs, the reader is advised to check the product information provided by the manufacturer of each drug for any change in dosages or for additional warnings and contraindications. This is of utmost importance when the recommended drug herein is a new or infrequently used drug. It is the responsibility of the treating physician to determine dosages and treatment strategies for individual patients. Further it is the responsibility of the health care provider to ascertain the Food and Drug Administration status of each drug or device used in their clinical practice. The publisher, editors, and authors are not responsible for errors or omissions or for any consequences from the application of the information presented in this book and make no warranty, express or implied, with respect to the contents in this publication.

This publication is printed on acid-free paper. ∞
ANSI Z39.48-1984 (American Standards Institute) Permanence of Paper for Printed Library Materials.

Production Editor: Robin B. Weisberg

Cover design by Patricia F. Cleary

or additional copies, pricing for bulk purchases, and/or information about other Humana titles, contact Humana at the above address or at any of the following numbers: Tel.: 973-256-1699; Fax: 973-256-8341; E-mail: orders@humanapr.com; or visit our Website: www.humanapress.com

Printed in the United States of America. 10 9 8 7 6 5 4 3 2 1

eISBN 1-59745-042-1

Library of Congress Cataloging-in-Publication Data

Hollenberg, Steven M.
   Cardiology in family practice : a practical guide / by Steven M. Hollenberg, Tracy Walker.
      p. ; cm. -- (Current clinical practice)
   Includes bibliographical references and index.
   ISBN 1-58829-509-5 (alk. paper)
   1. Cardiova£Ÿulaä[system--Diseases--Diagnosis. 2. Cardiovascular system--Diseases--
Treatment. 3. Family medicine.   I. Walker, Tracy, MD. II. Title. III. Series.
   [DNLM: 1. Cardiology--methods. 2. Cardiovascular Diseases
--diagnosis. 3. Cardiovascular Diseases--therapy. 4. Family Practice.
   WG 100 H737c 2006]
   RC669.H65 2006
   616.1--dc22   2005022679

Series Editor's Introduction

Family doctors see patients with cardiac risk factors and cardiac disease every single day, and each day they make decisions about the medical care of those patients. Over the last 20 years, there has been an explosion of knowledge and therapeutic choices for caring for patients with cardiac risk factors and disease. Heart disease accounts for 700,000 deaths per year in the United States, accounting for 28% of all annual deaths in the country *(1)*. In 2004, family doctors prescribed 29% of all cardiovascular drugs prescribed nationwide during approximately 70 million office visits *(2)*.

Cardiology in Family Practice: A Practical Guide by Drs. Steven Hollenberg and Tracy Walker is an erudite book that is unique for its short length combined with its breadth, covering the range of cardiovascular risk factors and disease that primary care physicians encounter in both inpatient and outpatient settings. The authors provide readers with information to competently care for patients and make clear diagnostic and therapeutic choices based on the best evidence currently available. They do this with a clarity of voice that is unusual in medical writing. *Cardiology in Family Practice: A Practical Guide* should be useful to all physicians in primary care who are looking to update their knowledge of cardiac disease, and who would like a concise, relevant textbook to read and to refer to on their shelves.

Neil Skolnik, MD
Associate Director
Family Medicine Residency Program
Abington Memorial Hospital
Professor of Family and Community Medicine
Temple University School of Medicine

REFERENCES

1. Cause of Death, US. National Center for Health Statistics, accessed September 13, 2005 at http://www.cdc.gov/nchs/data/dvs/LCWK1_2002.pdf
2. US Department of Health and Human Services, Public Health Service, Centers for Disease Control and Prevention, National Care for Health Statistics, 2002 data. Public Use data file. Accessed at http://www.aafp.org/x796.xml on September 13, 2005.

Preface

Cardiovascular disease (CVD) is an enormous problem in industrialized nations. Despite a declining incidence, an estimated 70 million Americans have some form of CVD, which causes more than 700,000 deaths and prompts 6.4 million hospital admissions each year. Given the aging of the population and the challenges in risk-factor management, these numbers are more likely to increase than decrease. In fact, better management of acute phases has led to an increased number of patients with chronic manifestations of CVD.

The response has been a prodigious effort on all fronts. Classic cardiovascular research encompasses physiology and pharmacology, but has now grown to include molecular biology, genetics, developmental biology, biophysics, bioengineering, and information technology, all of which are availing themselves of an impressive and ever-increasing set of sophisticated investigational tools. Old paradigms are under constant assault from a barrage of new information. Clinical research has developed just as quickly, generating a voluminous body of trial data that seems to grow exponentially.

All of this poses its own set of problems for practitioners, in particular those without subspecialty training in CVD. The rate of advance of clinical cardiology continues to accelerate, with new pathophysiological models, new imaging technologies, and new therapies. Meanwhile, the volume of cardiac patients, particularly in the hospital setting, is increasing.

With all of this in mind, we offer up this short volume, neither exhaustive nor all encompassing, but designed to be clear and concise. We hope to promote understanding of basic mechanisms underlying disease states because these provide the rationales for treatment strategies. The emphasis, however, is on delineating practical techniques for the evaluation and treatment of patients with cardiovascular problems. Along the same lines, references are not meant to be comprehensive, but to point the reader to the most useful sources of additional information. Our goal is to provide a fast and effective resource that will help practitioners to identify important concepts and information that they can use to deliver more effective patient care.

Steven M. Hollenberg, MD
Tracy Walker, MD

Contents

1 Acute Coronary Syndromes

TERMINOLOGY

Acute coronary syndromes (ACS) describe the spectrum of disease in patients who present with any constellation of clinical symptoms that are compatible with acute myocardial ischemia. ACS are a family of disorders that share similar pathogenic mechanisms and represent different points along a common continuum. These syndromes are caused by recent thrombus formation on pre-existing coronary artery plaque leading to impaired myocardial oxygen supply. In this sense, they differ from stable angina, which is usually precipitated by increased myocardial oxygen demand (e.g., exertion, fever, tachycardia) with background coronary artery narrowing (limitation of oxygen supply). (*See* Fig. 1.)

ACS have traditionally been classified into Q-wave myocardial infarction (MI), non-Q-wave myocardial infarction (NQMI), and unstable angina. More recently, classification has shifted and has become based on the initial electrocardiogram (ECG): patients are divided into three groups: those with ST-elevation MI (STEMI), without ST elevation but with enzyme evidence of myocardial damage (non-ST elevation MI [NSTEMI]), and those with unstable angina. Classification according to presenting ECG coincides with current treatment strategies because patients presenting with ST elevation benefit from immediate reperfusion and should be treated with thrombolytic therapy or urgent revascularization, whereas fibrinolytic agents are not effective in other patients with ACS. The discussion in this chapter follows this schematization.

Pathophysiology

The common link between the various ACS is the rupture of a vulnerable, but previously quiescent, coronary atherosclerotic plaque

From: *Current Clinical Practice: Cardiology in Family Practice:*
A Practical Guide
By: S. M. Hollenberg and T. Walker © Humana Press Inc., Totowa, NJ

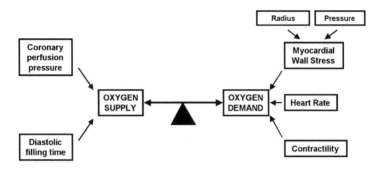

Fig. 1. Determinants of myocardial oxygen supply and demand.

(Libby, 2001). Exposure of plaque contents to the circulating blood pool triggers the release of vasoactive amines, and activation of platelets and the coagulation cascade. The extent of resultant platelet aggregation, thrombosis, vasoconstriction, and microembolization dictates the clinical manifestations of the syndrome. The relative fibrin and platelet content of these lesions vary, with unstable angina/NSTEMI more often associated with platelet-rich lesions and STEMI associated with fibrin-rich clot, although it should be noted that all lesions contain some degree of both components (Ambrose & Martinez, 2002). These observations form the scientific rationale for the use of fibrinolytic ("thrombolytic") agents in STEMI and platelet inhibitors in unstable angina/NSTEMI.

DIAGNOSIS

Signs and Symptoms

Patients with myocardial ischemia can present with chest pain or pressure, shortness of breath, palpitations, syncope, or sudden death. The pain of MI is typically severe, constant, and retrosternal. The pain commonly spreads across the chest and may radiate to the throat or jaw, or down the arms. Its duration is most often more than 20 minutes. Diaphoresis, nausea, pallor, and anxiety are often present. Prodromal symptoms of myocardial ischemia occur in 20 to 60% of patients in the days preceding the infarct. The pain of unstable angina may be similar, although it is often milder.

Although these are the classic signs of MI, it is important to recognize that the pain of MI may sometimes be atypical in terms of location or perception. It may be epigastric, confined to the jaw, arms, wrists or interscapular region, or perceived as burning or pressure.

The physical examination can be insensitive and nonspecific, but is useful in diagnosing specific complications and in excluding alternative diagnoses, both cardiovascular (such as aortic dissection or pericarditis) and non-cardiac. Distended jugular veins signal right ventricular diastolic pressure elevation, and the appearance of pulmonary crackles (in the absence of pulmonary disease) indicates elevated left ventricular (LV) filling pressures. LV failure is suggested by the presence of basal crackles, tachycardia and tachypnea, and an S3 gallop, which usually indicates a large infarction with extensive muscle damage. A systolic murmur of mitral regurgitation may be present owing to papillary muscle dysfunction or LV dilation. A pansystolic murmur may also result from an acute ventricular septal defect as a result of septal rupture.

The Electrocardiogram

The ECG abnormalities in myocardial ischemia depend on the extent and nature of coronary stenosis and the presence of collateral flow, but the pattern of ECG changes generally gives a guide to the area and extent of infarction (*see* Table 1). The number of leads involved broadly reflects the extent of myocardium involved.

With acute total acute occlusion of a coronary artery, the first demonstrable ECG changes are peaked T-waves changes in the leads reflecting the anatomic area of myocardium in jeopardy. As total occlusion continues, there is elevation of the ST segments in the same leads. With continued occlusion, there is an evolution of ECG abnormalities, with biphasic and then inverted T-waves. If enough myocardium is infarcted, Q-waves, which represent unopposed initial depolarization forces away from the mass of infarcted myocardium, which has lost electrical activity and no longer contributes to the mean QRS voltage vector, may appear. The formation of Q-waves is accompanied by a decrease in the magnitude of the R-waves in the same leads, representing diminution of voltage in the mass of infarcted myocardium. Indeed, loss of R-wave voltage, revealed by comparison with previous ECG tracings, may be the only ECG evidence for the presence of permanent myocardial damage.

Table 1
Localization of Myocardial Infarction by Electrocardiography

Area of infarction	ECG leads	Infarct-related artery
Inferior	II, III, aVF	RCA or posterolateral branch of Cx
Anterior	V2, V3, V4	LAD or Diagonal branch of LAD
Lateral	I, aVL, V5, V6	Cx
True posterior	Tall R wave in V1	Posterolateral branch of Cx or Posterior Descending Branch of RCA
Septal	V1-V3	LAD or Diagonal branch of LAD
Anterolateral	I, aVL, V2-V6	Proximal LAD
Inferolateral	II, III, aVF, I, aVL, V5, V6	Proximal Cx or large RCA in right dominant system
Right ventricular	V3R, V4R	RCA

RCA, right coronary artery; LAD, left anterior descending coronary artery; Cx, circumflex coronary artery.

Extension of an inferior MI to the posterior segment can be detected by enhancement of R-waves in the anterior chest leads because these forces are now less opposed by posterior forces. True posterior infarction can be subtle because the only signs may be prominent R-waves, tall upright T-waves and depressed ST segments in leads V_1 and V_2. Involvement of the right ventricle (RV) in inferior MI is also not readily detected on the standard 12-lead ECG because of the small mass of the RV relative to the LV and because of the positioning of the standard precordial leads away from the RV. RV infarction may be detected by ST elevation in recordings from right precordial leads, particularly V_{4R} (Croft et al., 1982).

The clinician must also be careful not to be fooled by ECG "imposters" of acute infarction, which include pericarditis, J-point elevation, Wolff-Parkinson-White syndrome, and hypertrophic cardiomyopathy. In pericarditis, ST segments may be elevated, but the elevation is diffuse and the morphology of the ST segments in pericarditis tends to be concave upward, whereas that of ischemia is convex. Pericarditis may also be distinguished from infarction by the presence of PR segment depression in the inferior leads (and also by PR segment in lead aVR) (Spodick, 1973).

Cardiac Biomarkers

Measurement of enzymes released into the serum from necrotic myocardial cells after infarction can aid in the diagnosis of MI (Lee & Goldman, 1986; Rapaport, 1977). The classic biochemical marker of acute MI is elevation of the creatine phosphokinase (CPK) MB isoenzyme. CPK MB begins to appear in the plasma 4 to 8 hours after onset of infarction, peaks at 12 to 24 hours and returns to baseline at 2 to 4 days. To be diagnostic for MI, the total plasma CPK value must exceed the upper limit of normal, and the MB fraction must exceed a certain value (usually >5%, but depends on the CPK MB assay used).

A newer serological test for the detection of myocardial damage employs measurement of cardiac troponins (Katus et al., 1991). Troponin T and troponin I are constituents of the contractile protein apparatus of cardiac muscle. Whereas CPK MB may arise from other tissues, troponins originate only from cardiac muscle, rendering them more specific than the conventional CPK MB assays for the detection of myocardial damage. Their use is becoming more widespread, and has superceded the use of CPK MB in many settings (Jaffe et al., 2000). Troponins are also more sensitive for the detection of myocardial damage, and troponin elevation in patients without ST elevation (or, in fact, without elevation of CPK MB) identifies a subpopulation at increased risk for complications. Rapid point-of-care troponin assays, which have become available in the past few years, have further extended the clinical utility of this marker. Troponins may not be elevated until 6 hours after an acute event, and so critical therapeutic interventions should not be delayed pending assay results. Once elevated, troponin levels can remain high for days to weeks, limiting their utility to detect late reinfarction.

ST ELEVATION MYOCARDIAL INFARCTION

Symptoms suggestive of MI are usually similar to those of ordinary angina but are greater in intensity and duration. Nausea, vomiting, and diaphoresis may be prominent features, and stupor and malaise attributable to low cardiac output may occur. Compromised LV function may result in pulmonary edema with development of pulmonary bibasilar crackles and jugular venous distention; a fourth heart sound can be present with small infarcts or even mild ischemia, but a third heart sound is usually indicative of more extensive damage.

Patients presenting with suspected myocardial ischemia should undergo a rapid evaluation, and should be treated with oxygen, sublingual nitroglycerin (unless systolic blood pressure is less than 90 mmHg), adequate analgesia, and aspirin, 160 to 325 mg orally (Ryan et al., 1999). Narcotics should be used to relieve pain, and also reduce anxiety, the salutary effects of which have been known for decades and must not be underestimated. It is also important to provide reassurance to the patient. A 12-lead ECG should be performed and interpreted expeditiously.

ST-segment elevation of at least 1 mV in two or more contiguous leads provides strong evidence of thrombotic coronary occlusion. The patient should be considered for immediate reperfusion therapy. The diagnosis of STEMI can be limited in the presence of pre-existing left bundle branch block (LBBB) or permanent pacemaker. Nonetheless, new LBBB with a compatible clinical presentation should be treated as acute MI and treated accordingly. Indeed, recent data suggest that patients with STEMI and new LBBB may stand to gain greater benefit from reperfusion strategies than those with ST elevation and preserved ventricular conduction.

Thrombolytic Therapy

Early reperfusion of an occluded coronary artery is indicated for all eligible candidates. Overwhelming evidence from multiple clinical trials demonstrates the ability of thrombolytic agents administered early in the course of an acute MI to reduce infarct size, preserve LV function, and reduce short- and long-term mortality (Gruppo Italiano per lo Studio della Streptochinasi nell'Infarto Miocardico [GISSI], 1986; Thrombolysis in Myocardial Infarction [TIMI] Study Group, 1985). Patients treated early derive the most benefit. Indications and contraindications for thrombolytic therapy are listed in Table 2. Because of the small, but nonetheless significant, risk of a bleeding complication, most notably intracranial hemorrhage (ICH), selection of patients with acute MI for administration of a thrombolytic agent

Table 2
Indications for and Contraindications
to Thrombolytic Therapy in Acute Myocardial Infarction

Indications

- Symptoms consistent with acute myocardial infarction
- ECG showing 1-mm (0.1 mV) ST elevation in at least two contiguous leads, or new left bundle branch block
- Presentation within 12 hours of symptom onset
- Absence of contraindications

Contraindications

Absolute

- Active internal bleeding
- Intracranial neoplasm, aneurysm, or AV malformation
- Stroke or neurosurgery within 6 weeks
- Trauma or major surgery within 2 weeks, which could be a potential source of serious rebleeding
- Aortic dissection

Relative

- Prolonged (>10 minutes) or clearly traumatic cardiopulmonary resuscitation[a]
- Noncompressible vascular punctures
- Severe uncontrolled hypertension (>200/110 mmHg)[a]
- Trauma or major surgery within 6 weeks (but >2 weeks)
- Pre-existing coagulopathy or current use of anticoagulants with INR >2–3
- Active peptic ulcer
- Infective endocarditis
- Pregnancy
- Chronic severe hypertension

[a] Could be an absolute contraindication in low-risk patients with myocardial infarction. ECG, electrocardiogram; AV, arterioventricular; INR, international normalized ratio.

should be undertaken with prudence and caution. Some patients may be better treated with emergent coronary angiography with percutaneous coronary intervention (PCI) as clinically indicated.

In contrast to the treatment of STEMI, thrombolytics have shown no benefit to increased risk of adverse events when used for the treatment of unstable angina/NSTEMI (TIMI Investigators, 1994).

Based on these findings, there is currently no role for thrombolytic agents in these latter syndromes.

THROMBOLYTIC AGENTS

Streptokinase (SK) is a single-chain protein produced by α-hemolytic streptococci. SK is given as a 1.5 million unit intravenous infusion over 1 hour, which produces a systemic lytic state for about 24 hours. Hypotension with infusion usually responds to fluids and a decreased infusion rate, but allergic reactions are possible. Hemorrhagic complications are the most feared side effect, with a rate of ICH of approximately 0.5%. SK produces coronary arterial patency approximately 50 to 60% of the time, and has been shown to decrease mortality 18% compared with placebo (GISSI, 1986).

Tissue plasminogen activator (t-PA) is a recombinant protein that is more fibrin-selective than SK and produces a higher early coronary patency rate (70–80%). In the large (41,021 patients) Global Utilization of Streptokinase and Tissue Plasminogen Activator for Occluded Coronary Arteries (GUSTO) trial, t-PA demonstrated a small but significant survival benefit compared with SK in patients with STEMI (1.1% absolute, 15% relative reduction) (GUSTO Investigators, 1993). The GUSTO angiographic substudy showed that the difference in patency rates explains the difference in clinical efficacy between these two agents (GUSTO Angiographic Investigators, 1993). t-PA is usually given in an accelerated regimen consisting of a 15 mg bolus, 0.75 mg/kg (up to 50 mg) intravenously over the initial 30 minutes, and 0.5 mg/kg (up to 35 mg) over the next 60 minutes. Allergic reactions do not occur because t-PA is not antigenic, but the rate of ICH may be slightly higher than that with SK, around 0.7%.

Reteplase (r-PA) is a deletion mutant of t-PA with an extended half-life, and is given as two 10 mg boluses 30 minutes apart. r-PA was originally evaluated in angiographic trials that demonstrated improved coronary flow at 90 minutes compared with t-PA, but subsequent trials showed similar 30-day mortality rates (GUSTO III Investigators, 1997). Why enhanced patency with r-PA did not translate into lower mortality is uncertain.

Tenecteplase (TNK-tPA) is a genetically engineered t-PA mutant with amino acid substitutions that result in prolonged half-life, resistance to plasminogen-activator inhibitor-1, and increased fibrin specificity. TNK-tPA is given as a single bolus, adjusted for weight.

A single bolus of TNK-tPA has been shown to produced coronary flow rates identical to those seen with accelerated t-PA, with equivalent 30-day mortality and bleeding rates (Assessment of the Safety and Efficacy of a New Thrombolytic Investigators, 1999). Based on these results, single-bolus TNK-tPA is an acceptable alternative to t-PA that can be given as a single bolus.

Because these newer agents in general have equivalent efficacy and side effect profiles, at no current additional cost compared to t-PA, and because they are simpler to administer, they have gained popularity. The ideal thrombolytic agent has not yet been developed. Newer recombinant agents with greater fibrin specificity, slower clearance from the circulation, and more resistance to plasma protease inhibitors are being studied.

Primary Percutaneous Coronary Intervention in Acute Myocardial Infarction

As many as 50 to 66% of patients presenting with acute MI may be ineligible for thrombolytic therapy, and these patients should be considered for primary PCI. The major advantages of primary PCI over thrombolytic therapy include a higher rate of normal (TIMI grade 3) (TIMI Study Group, 1985) flow, lower risk of ICH and the ability to stratify risk based on the severity and distribution of coronary artery disease (CAD). Data from several randomized trials have suggested that PCI is preferable to thrombolytic therapy for acute MI patients at higher risk, including those over 75 years old, those with anterior infarctions, and those with hemodynamic instability (Grines et al., 1993). The largest of these trials is the GUSTO-IIb Angioplasty Substudy, which randomized 1138 patients. At 30 days, there was a clinical benefit in the combined primary endpoints of death, nonfatal reinfarction, and nonfatal disabling stroke in the patients treated with percutaneous transluminal coronary angioplasty (PTCA) compared with t-PA, but no difference in the "hard" endpoints of death and MI at 30 days (GUSTO IIb Investigators, 1996).

It should be noted that these trials were performed in institutions in which a team skilled in primary angioplasty for acute MI was immediately available, with standby surgical backup, allowing for prompt reperfusion of the infarct-related artery. More important than the method of revascularization is the time to revascularization, and that this should be achieved in the most efficient and expeditious manner possible (Cannon et al., 2000). Procedural volume is important as well (Canto et al., 2000). A recent meta-analysis comparing direct PTCA with thrombolytic therapy found lower rates of mortality and reinfarction among those receiving direct PTCA (Grines et al., 2003; Keeley et al., 2003). Thus, direct angioplasty, if performed in a timely manner (ideally within 60 minutes) by highly experienced personnel, may be the preferred method of revascularization because it offers more complete revascularization with improved restoration of normal coronary blood flow and detailed information about coronary anatomy.

Historically, it has been felt that when performing PCI will require a substantial time delay, thrombolytic therapy may be preferable. Recently reported studies comparing in-house thrombolysis to hospital transfer for PCI have challenged this notion, however. In the PRAGUE-2 study, there was no difference in mortality between patients treated within 3 hours either with thrombolysis using SK or off-site PCI (Widimsky et al., 2003). Interestingly, in patients treated between 3 and 12 hours, transfer for PCI conferred significant mortality benefit despite adding to the time to treatment (Widimsky et al., 2003). Similar results were found in DANAMI-2, in which referral for primary PCI reducing the occurrence of a composite endpoint of death, reinfarction or stroke, compared with thrombolysis using t-PA (Andersen et al., 2003). Although these data are intriguing, the importance of procedural volume and experience has been underscored by retrospective studies which have suggested that in the community setting (as opposed to PCI performed as part of a controlled clinical trial), mortality rates after MI with routine primary PCI and thrombolytic therapy are currently equivalent. More controversial is the issue of performing PCI at centers without onsite surgical backup. Although emerging data suggest that is practice is not only feasible but also safe (Aversano et al., 2002), further large-scale investigations will be necessary to clarify this issue.

There are certain subpopulations in which primary PCI is preferred. In patients who fail thrombolytic therapy, salvage PTCA is indicated, although the initial success rate is lower than that of primary angioplasty, reocclusion is more common, and mortality is higher. The RESCUE trial focused on a subset of acute MI patients

Table 3
Situations in Which Primary Angioplasty
is Preferred in Acute Myocardial Infarction

Situations in which PTCA is clearly preferable to thrombolytics
- Contraindications to thrombolytic therapy
- Cardiogenic shock
- Patients in whom uncertain diagnosis prompted cardiac catheterization that revealed coronary occlusion

Situations in which PTCA may be preferable to thrombolytics
- Elderly patients (>75 years)
- Hemodynamic instability
- Patients with prior coronary artery bypass grafting
- Large anterior infarction
- Patients with a prior myocardial infarction

with anterior infarction and showed a reduction in the combined endpoint of death or congestive heart failure at 30 days in the group receiving salvage PTCA (Ellis et al., 1994). Emergent cardiac catheterization is also preferred in patients with cardiogenic shock. Other indications are listed in Table 3.

There is no convincing evidence to support empirical delayed PTCA in patients without evidence of recurrent or provokable ischemia after thrombolytic therapy. The TIMI IIB trial and others studies suggest that a strategy of "watchful waiting" allows for identification of patients who will benefit from revascularization (TIMI Study Group, 1989).

Adjunctive Therapies in STEMI

ASPIRIN

Aspirin has been shown to reduce mortality in acute MI to the same degree as thrombolytic therapy, and its effects are additive to thrombolytics (ISIS-2 [Second International Study of Infarct Survival] Collaborative Group, 1988). In addition, aspirin reduces the risk of reinfarction. Unless contraindicated, all patients with a suspected ACS (STEMI, NSTEMI, unstable angina) should be given aspirin as soon as possible.

HEPARIN

Administration of full-dose heparin after thrombolytic therapy with t-PA is essential to diminish reocclusion after successful reperfusion (GISSI, 1986; ISIS-2, 1988) Dosing should be adjusted to weight, with a bolus of 60 U/kg up to a maximum of 4000 U and an initial infusion rate of 12 U/kg per hour up to a maximum of 1000 U per hour, with adjustment to keep the partial thromboplastin time between 50 and 70 seconds. Heparin should be continued for 24 to 48 hours.

NITRATES

Nitrates have a number of beneficial effects in acute MI. They reduce myocardial oxygen demand by decreasing preload and afterload, and may also improve myocardial oxygen supply by increasing subendocardial perfusion and collateral blood flow to the ischemic region. Occasional patients with ST elevation as a result of occlusive coronary artery spasm may have dramatic resolution of ischemia with nitrates. In addition to their hemodynamic effects, nitrates also reduce platelet aggregation. Despite these benefits, the GISSI-3 and ISIS-4 trials failed to show a significant reduction in mortality from routine acute and chronic nitrate therapy (GISSI, 1994; ISIS-4 (Fourth International Study of Infarct Survival) Study Group, 1995) Nonetheless, nitrates are still first-line agents for the symptomatic relief of angina pectoris and when MI is complicated by congestive heart failure.

β-BLOCKERS

β-blockers are beneficial both in the early management of MI and as long-term therapy. In the pre-thrombolytic era, early intravenous atenolol was shown to significantly reduce reinfarction, cardiac arrest, cardiac rupture, and death (First International Study of Infarct Survival Collaborative Group, 1986). In conjunction with thrombolytic therapy with t-PA, immediate β-blockade with metoprolol resulted in a significant reduction in recurrent ischemia and reinfarction, although mortality was not decreased (TIMI Study Group, 1989).

Administration of intravenous β-blockade should be considered for all patients presenting with acute MI, especially those with continued ischemic discomfort and sympathetic hyperactivity manifested by hypertension or tachycardia. Therapy should be avoided in patients with moderate or severe heart failure, hypotension, severe bradycardia or heart block, and severe bronchospastic disease. Metoprolol can be given as a 5 mg intravenous bolus, repeated every 5 minutes for a total of three doses. Because of its brief half-life, esmolol may be advantageous in situations were precise control or the heart rate is necessary or rapid drug withdrawal may be needed if adverse effects occur.

Oral β-blockade has been clearly demonstrated to decrease mortality after acute MI (Dargie, 2001; The International Collaborative Study Group, 1984; MIAMI Trial Research Group, 1985), and should be initiated in all patients who can tolerate it, even if they have not been treated with intravenous β-blockers. Diabetes mellitus is not a contraindication.

Lipid-Lowering Agents

There is extensive epidemiological, laboratory, and clinical evidence linking cholesterol and CAD. Total cholesterol level has been linked to the development of CAD events with a continuous and graded relation (Lipid Research Clinics Program, 1984). Most of this risk is caused by low-density lipoprotein cholesterol (LDL-C). A number of large primary and secondary prevention trials have shown that LDL-C lowering is associated with a reduced risk of CAD events. Earlier lipid-lowering trials used bile-acid sequestrants (cholestyramine), fibric acid derivatives (gemfibrozil and clofibrate), or niacin in addition to diet. The reduction in total cholesterol in these early trials was 6 to 15% and was accompanied by a consistent trend toward a reduction in fatal and nonfatal coronary events (Frick et al., 1987).

More impressive results have been achieved using hydroxymethylglutaryl coenzyme A reductase inhibitors (statins). Statins have been demonstrated to decrease the rate of adverse ischemic events in patients with documented CAD in the 4S trial (Scandinavian Simvastatin Survival Study Group, 1994) as well as in the CARE study (Sacks et al., 1996) and the LIPID trial (Long-Term Intervention with Pravastatin in Ischaemic Disease [LIPID] Study Group, 1998).

The goal of treatment is an LDL-C level less than 70 to 100 mg/dL (Gibbons et al., 2003). Maximum benefit may require management of other lipid abnormalities (elevated triglycerides, low high-density lipoprotein cholesterol) and treatment of other atherogenic risk factors.

ANGIOTENSIN-CONVERTING ENZYME INHIBITORS

Angiotensin-converting enzyme (ACE) inhibitors are clearly beneficial in patients with congestive heart failure. ACE inhibitors were shown to decrease mortality in the SAVE trial, in which patients with LV dysfunction (ejection fraction <40%) after MI had a 21% improvement in survival after treatment with the ACE inhibitor captopril (Pfeffer et al., 1992). A smaller but still significant reduction in mortality was seen when all patients were treated with captopril in the ISIS-4 study (ISIS-4, 1995). The mechanisms responsible for the benefits of ACE inhibitors probably include limitation in the progressive LV dysfunction and enlargement (remodeling) that often occur after infarction, but a reduction in ischemic events was seen as well.

ACE inhibition should be started early, preferably within the first 24 hours after MI. Immediate intravenous ACE inhibition with enalaprilat has not been shown to be beneficial (Edner et al., 1996). Patients should be started on low doses of oral agents (captopril 6.25 mg three times daily) and rapidly increased to the range demonstrated beneficial in clinical trials (captopril 50 mg three times daily, enalapril 10 to 20 mg twice daily, lisinopril 10 to 20 mg once daily, or ramipril 10 mg once daily).

CALCIUM CHANNEL BLOCKERS

Randomized clinical trials have not demonstrated that routine use of calcium channel blockers (CCBs) improves survival after MI. In fact, meta-analyses suggest that high doses of the short-acting dihydropyridine nifedipine increase mortality in MI. Adverse effects of CCBs include bradycardia, atrioventricular block, and exacerbation of heart failure. The relative vasodilating, negative inotropic effects, and conduction system effects of the various agents must be considered when they are employed in this setting. Diltiazem is the only CCB that has been proven to have tangible benefits, reducing reinfarction and recurrent ischemia in patients with patients with non-Q-wave infarctions who do not have evidence of congestive heart failure (Gibson et al., 1986).

CCBs may be useful for patients whose postinfarction course is complicated by recurrent angina, because these agents not only reduce myocardial oxygen demand but inhibit coronary vasocon-striction. For hemodynamically stable patients, diltiazem can be given, starting at 60 to 90 mg orally every 6 to 8 hours. In patients with severe LV dysfunction, long-acting dihydropyridines without prominent negative inotropic effects such as amlodipine, nicardi-pine, or the long-acting preparation of nifedipine may be preferable; increased mortality with these agents has not been demonstrated.

Antiarrhythmic Therapy

A major purpose for admitting MI patients to the intensive care unit is to monitor for and prevent malignant arrhythmias. Ventricular extrasystoles are common after MI and are a manifestation of elec-trical instability of peri-infarct areas. The incidence of sustained ventricular tachycardia or fibrillation is highest in the first 3 to 4 hours, but these arrhythmias may occur at any time. Malignant ven-tricular arrhythmias may be heralded by frequent premature ven-tricular contractions (PVCs) (more than five or six per minute), closely coupled PVCs, complex ectopy (couplets, multiform PVCs) and salvos of nonsustained ventricular tachycardia. However, malig-nant arrhythmia may occur suddenly without these preceding "warn-ing" arrhythmias. Based on these pathophysiological considerations, prophylactic use of intravenous lidocaine even in the absence of ectopy has been advocated.

Although lidocaine increases the frequency of PVCs and of early ventricular fibrillation, overall mortality is not decreased. In fact, meta-analyses of pooled data have demonstrated increased mortal-ity from the routine use of lidocaine (MacMahon et al., 1988). There-fore, routine prophylactic administration of lidocaine is no longer recommended.

Nonetheless, lidocaine infusion may be useful after an episode of sustained ventricular tachycardia or ventricular fibrillation, and could be considered in patients with nonsustained ventricular tachycardia. Lidocaine is administered as a bolus of 1 mg/kg (not to exceed 100 mg), followed by a second bolus of 0.5 mg/kg 10 minutes later, along with an infusion at 1 to 3 mg per minute. Lidocaine is metabolized by the liver, and so lower doses should be given in the presence of liver disease, in the elderly, and in patients who have congestive heart failure severe enough to compromise hepatic perfusion. Toxic manifestations primarily involve the central nervous system, and can include confusion, lethargy, slurred speech, and seizures. Because the risk of malignant ventricular arrhythmias decreases after 24 hours, lidocaine is usually discontinued after this point. For prolonged infusions, monitoring of lidocaine levels (therapeutic between 1.5 and 5 g/mL) is sometimes useful.

Intravenous amiodarone is an alternative to lidocaine for ventricular arrhythmias. Amiodarone is given as a 150 mg intravenous bolus over 10 minutes, followed by 1 mg per minute for 6 hours, then 0.5 mg per minute for 18 hours.

Perhaps the most important point in the prevention and management of arrhythmias after acute MI is correcting hypoxemia, and maintaining normal serum potassium and magnesium levels. Serum electrolytes should be followed closely, particularly after diuretic therapy. Magnesium depletion is also a frequently overlooked cause of persistent ectopy (Lauler, 1989). The serum magnesium level, even if it is within normal limits, may not reflect myocardial concentrations. Routine administration of magnesium has not been shown to reduce mortality after acute MI (ISIS-4, 1995) but empiric administration of 2 g of intravenous magnesium in patients with early ventricular ectopy is probably a good idea.

One possible treatment algorithm for treating patients with STEMI is shown in Fig. 2.

NON-ST ELEVATION MYOCARDIAL INFARCTION

The key to initial management of patients with ACS who present without ST elevation is risk stratification. The overall risk of a patient is related to both the severity of pre-existing heart disease and the degree of plaque instability. Risk stratification is an ongoing process that begins with hospital admission and continues through discharge.

Braunwald (1989) proposed a classification for unstable angina based on severity of symptoms and clinical circumstances for risk stratification. The risk of progression to acute MI or death in ACS increases with age. ST-segment depression on the ECG identifies patients at higher risk for clinical events (Braunwald, 1989). Conversely, a normal ECG confers an excellent short-term prognosis. Biochemical markers of cardiac injury are also predictive of outcome. Elevated levels of troponin T are associated with an increased

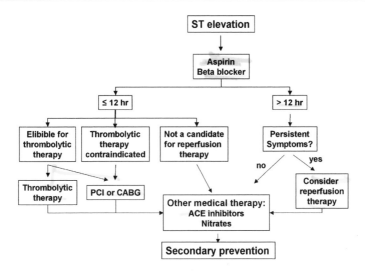

Fig. 2. Possible treatment algorithm for patients presenting with ST elevation myocardial infarction. PCI, percutaneous coronary intervention; CABG, coronary artery bypass grafting; ACE, angiotensin-converting enzyme.

risk of cardiac events and a higher 30-day mortality, and in fact, were more strongly correlated with 30-day survival than ECG category or CPK MB level in an analysis of data from the GUSTO-2 trial (Ohman et al., 1996). Conversely, low levels are associated with low event rates, although the absence of troponin elevation does not guarantee a good prognosis and is not a substitute for good clinical judgment.

Antiplatelet Therapy

As previously noted, aspirin is a mainstay of therapy for ACS. Both the VA Cooperative Study Group (Lewis et al., 1983) and the Canadian Multicenter Trial (Cairns et al., 1985) showed that aspirin reduces the risk of death or MI by approximately 50% in patients with unstable angina or NQMI. Aspirin also reduces events after resolution of an ACS, and should be continued indefinitely.

Clopidogrel or ticlopidine, thienopyridines that inhibit adenosine diphosphate-induced platelet activation and are more potent than aspirin, can be used in place of aspirin if necessary. They are used in combination with aspirin when intracoronary stents are placed. Clopidogrel is generally better tolerated than ticlopidine because the risk of neutropenia is much lower.

Clopidogrel added to aspirin significantly reduced the risk of MI, stroke, or cardiovascular death from 11.4 to 9.3% ($p < 0.001$) in 12,562 patients with unstable angina in the randomized CURE trial (Yusuf et al., 2001). It should be noted that this benefit came with a 1% absolute increase in major, bleeds ($p = 0.001$) as well as a 2.8% absolute increase in major/life-threatening bleeds associated with coronary artery bypass graft (CABG) within 5 days ($p = 0.07$) (Yusuf et al., 2001). These data have raised concerns about giving clopidogrel prior to information about the coronary anatomy. Clopidogrel has also been tested for secondary prevention of events (CAPRIE Steering Committee, 1996).

Anticoagulant Therapy

Heparin is an important component of primary therapy for patients with unstable coronary syndromes without ST elevation. When added to aspirin, heparin has been shown to reduce refractory angina and the development of MI (Theroux et al., 1988), and a meta-analysis of the available data indicates that addition of heparin reduces the composite endpoint of death or MI (Oler et al., 1996).

Heparin, however, can be difficult to administer, because the anticoagulant effect is unpredictable in individual patients; this is due to heparin binding to heparin-binding proteins, endothelial and other cells, and heparin inhibition by several factors released by activated platelets. Therefore, the activated partial thromboplastin time (APTT) must be monitored closely. The potential for heparin-associated thrombocytopenia is also a safety concern.

Low-molecular-weight heparins (LMWH), which are obtained by depolymerization of standard heparin and selection of fractions with lower molecular weight, have several advantages. Because they bind less avidly to heparin-binding proteins, there is less variability in the anticoagulant response and a more predictable dose–response curve, obviating the need to monitor APTT. The incidence of thrombocytopenia is lower (but not absent, and patients with heparin-induced thrombocytopenia with anti-heparin antibodies cannot be switched to LMWH). Finally, LMWHs have longer half-lives, and can be given by subcutaneous injection.

Several trials have documented beneficial effects of LMWH therapy in unstable coronary syndromes. The ESSENCE and TIMI 11B trials showed that the LMWH enoxaparin reduced the combined endpoint of death, MI, or recurrent ischemia compared with unfractionated heparin (UFH). Similar results were found in the TIMI 11B trial comparing enoxaparin to heparin (Antman et al., 1999). The recent SYNERGY trial found no difference in efficacy between enoxaparin and UFH in high-risk patients, with a slightly higher major bleeding rate (Ferguson et al., 2004). Specific considerations with the use of LMWH include decreased clearance in renal insufficiency and the lack of a commercially available test to measure the anticoagulant effect. LMWH is a safe and effective alternative to UFH, but the advantages of convenience should be balanced against a modest excess of major bleeding and cost considerations.

Glycoprotein IIb/IIIa Antagonists

Given the central role of platelet activation and aggregation in the pathophysiology of unstable coronary syndromes, attention has focused on platelet glycoprotein (GP) IIb/IIIa antagonists, which inhibit the final common pathway of platelet aggregation (Chew & Moliterno, 2000). Three agents are currently available: abciximab, a chimeric murine-human monoclonal antibody Fab fragment; eptifibatide, a small molecule cyclic heptapeptide; and tirofiban, a small molecule, synthetic nonpeptide agent. The benefits of GP IIb/IIIa inhibitors as adjunctive treatment in patients undergoing PCI have been substantial and consistently observed (Chew & Moliterno, 2000). Abciximab has been most extensively studied, but a benefit for eptifibatide has also been demonstrated.

In ACS, the evidence supporting the efficacy of GP IIb/IIIa inhibitors is somewhat less impressive. Five major trials have been completed (the "4 Ps" and GUSTO-IV). In the Platelet Receptor Inhibition in Ischemic Syndrome Management (PRISM) trial, tirofiban reduced death, MI, or refractory ischemia when compared with heparin from 5.6 to 3.8% ($p < 0.01$) at 48 hours, but there was no difference at 30 days (7.1 versus 5.8%, $p = 0.11$) (PRISM Study Investigators, 1998). In the subsequent PRISM-PLUS trial, tirofiban added to heparin reduced death, MI, or refractory ischemia at 30 days from 11.9 to 8.7% ($p = 0.03$) (PRISM-PLUS Study Investigators, 1998). In the PURSUIT trial, eptifibatide reduced the rate of death or MI from 15.7 to 14.2% ($p = 0.04$) at 30 days (The PURSUIT Trial Investigators, 1998). The PARAGON trial with lamifiban did not show a significant benefit with GP IIb/IIIa inhibition (PARAGON Investigators, 1998). In the GUSTO-IV ACS trial, however, abciximab did not produce an improvement; in fact, death or MI was slightly higher with in the treatment group (Simoons, 2001). This trial included patients for whom PCI was not planned; when patients with refractory angina and planned angioplasty were randomized to receive abciximab or placebo from 24 hours prior to the procedure through 1 hour following PTCA in the CAPTURE (1997) trial, the primary endpoint, death, MI, or urgent revascularization at 30 days, was reduced by GP IIb/IIIa inhibition, and the rate of MI before PTCA was reduced as well (CAPTURE Investigators, 1997). When patients were broken down into those with and without increased troponin, the benefit was confined to the positive troponin group (CAPTURE Investigators, 1997).

Recent meta-analyses have found a relative risk reduction of 40% for GP IIb/IIIa therapy adjunctive to PCI, and a reduction of 11% for GP IIb/IIIa inhibitors in NSTEMI ACS (Chew & Moliterno, 2000). Additional analysis suggests that GP IIb/IIIa inhibition is most effective in high-risk patients, those with either ECG changes or elevated troponin (Chew & Moliterno, 2000). The benefits appear to accrue primarily in patients undergoing PCI, which may not be entirely surprising.

Interventional Management

Cardiac catheterization may be undertaken in patients presenting with symptoms suggestive of unstable coronary syndromes for one of several reasons: to assist with risk stratification, as a prelude to revascularization, and to exclude significant epicardial coronary stenosis as a cause of symptoms when the diagnosis is uncertain.

An early invasive approach has now been compared to a conservative approach in several prospective studies. Two earlier trials, the TIMI IIIb study (TIMI Investigators, 1994) and the VANQWISH trial (Boden et al., 1998) were negative. These trials were performed before widespread use of coronary stenting and platelet GP IIb/IIIa inhibitors, both of which have now been shown to improve outcomes after angioplasty. In addition, the crossover rate in the TIMI

IIIb study was high, and the VANQWISH study had a very high surgical mortality.

More recently, a substudy of FRISC II randomized 2457 patients to an early invasive or noninvasive strategy, and found a significantly lower 30-day mortality with an interventional approach, which was maintained at 1 year (FRISC II, 1999). The TACTICS TIMI-18 trial of 2220 patients found a significant reduction in the combined endpoint of death, MI, or re-admission for ACS with invasive management (Cannon et al., 2001). It is important to recognize that both of these trials selected high-risk patients (identified either on the basis of ECG changes or enzyme elevations) for inclusion. Addition of adjunctive antiplatelet therapy beyond the use of aspirin alone in conjunction with reperfusion may also have contributed to the improved outcomes with invasive strategies in these more recent trials.

Risk stratification is the key to managing patients with NSTEMI ACS. One possible algorithm for managing patients with NSTEMI is shown in Fig. 3. An initial strategy of medical management with attempts at stabilization is warranted in patients with lower risk, but patients at higher risk should be considered for cardiac catheterization. Pharmacological and mechanical strategies are intertwined in the sense that selection of patients for early revascularization will influence the choice of antiplatelet and anticoagulant medication. When good clinical judgment is employed, early coronary angiography in selected patients with ACS can lead to better management and lower morbidity and mortality.

COMPLICATIONS OF ACUTE
MYOCARDIAL INFARCTION
Postinfarction Ischemia

Ischemia after MI can be the result of mechanical problems that increase myocardial oxygen demand, and extracardiac factors such as hypertension, anemia, hypotension, or hypermetabolic states, but it usually results from decreased myocardial oxygen supply owing to coronary reocclusion or spasm. Immediate management includes aspirin, β-blockade, intravenous nitroglycerin, heparin, consideration of CCBs, and diagnostic coronary angiography. Post-infarction angina is an indication for revascularization. PTCA can be

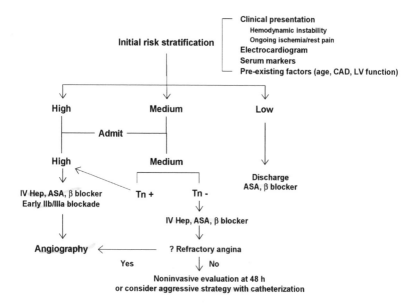

Fig. 3. Possible treatment algorithm for patients with non-ST elevation acute coronary syndromes. IV, intravenous; Hep, heparin; ASA, aspirin; Tn, troponin.

performed if the culprit lesion is suitable. CABG should be considered for patients with left main disease, three-vessel disease, and those unsuitable for PTCA. If the angina cannot be controlled medically or is accompanied by hemodynamic instability, an intra-aortic balloon pump (IABP) should be inserted.

Ventricular Free Wall Rupture

Ventricular free wall rupture typically occurs during the first week after MI. The classic patient is elderly, female, and hypertensive. Early use of thrombolytic therapy reduces the incidence of cardiac rupture, but late use may actually increase the risk. Free wall rupture presents as a catastrophic event with shock and electromechanical dissociation. Salvage is possible with prompt recognition, pericardiocentesis to relieve acute tamponade, and thoracotomy with repair (Reardon et al., 1997). Emergent echocardiography or pulmonary artery catheterization can help make the diagnosis.

Ventricular Septal Rupture

Septal rupture presents as severe heart failure or cardiogenic shock, with a pansystolic murmur and parasternal thrill. The hallmark finding is a left-to-right intracardiac shunt ("step-up" in oxygen saturation from right atrium to RV), but the diagnosis is most easily made with echocardiography.

Rapid institution of IABP and supportive pharmacological measures is necessary. Operative repair is the only viable option for long-term survival. The timing of surgery has been controversial, but most authorities now suggest that repair should be undertaken early, within 48 hours of the rupture (Killen et al., 1997).

Acute Mitral Regurgitation

Ischemic mitral regurgitation is usually associated with inferior MI and ischemia or infarction of the posterior papillary muscle, although anterior papillary muscle rupture can also occur. Papillary muscle rupture typically occurs 2 to 7 days after acute MI and presents dramatically with pulmonary edema, hypotension, and cardiogenic shock. When a papillary muscle ruptures, the murmur of acute mitral regurgitation may be limited to early systole because of rapid equalization of pressures in the left atrium and left ventricle. More importantly, the murmur may be soft or inaudible, especially when cardiac output is low (Khan & Gray, 1991).

Echocardiography is extremely useful in the differential diagnosis, which includes free wall rupture, ventricular septal rupture, and infarct extension with pump failure. Hemodynamic monitoring with pulmonary artery catheterization may also be helpful. Management includes afterload reduction with nitroprusside and IABP as temporizing measures. Inotropic or vasopressor therapy may also be needed to support cardiac output and blood pressure. Definitive therapy, however, is surgical valve repair or replacement, which should be undertaken as soon as possible because clinical deterioration can be sudden (Bolooki, 1989; Khan & Gray, 1991).

Right Ventricular Infarction

RV infarction occurs in up to 30% of patients with inferior MI and is clinically significant in 10% (Zehender et al., 1993). The combination of a clear chest x-ray with jugular venous distention in a patient with an inferior wall MI should lead to the suspicion of a co-existing RV infarct. The diagnosis is substantiated by demonstration of ST segment elevation in the right precordial leads (V_{3R} to V_{5R}) or by characteristic hemodynamic findings on right heart catheterization (elevated right atrial and RV end-diastolic pressures with normal to low pulmonary artery occlusion pressure and low cardiac output). Echocardiography can demonstrate depressed RV contractility (Kinch & Ryan, 1994). Patients with cardiogenic shock on the basis of RV infarction have a better prognosis than those with left-sided pump failure (Zehender et al., 1993). This may in part be the result of the fact that RV function tends to return to normal over time with supportive therapy (Dell'Italia et al., 1985), although such therapy may need to be prolonged.

In patients with RV infarction, RV preload should be maintained with fluid administration. In some cases, however, fluid resuscitation may increase pulmonary capillary occlusion pressure but may not increase cardiac output, and overdilation of the right ventricle can compromise LV filling and cardiac output (Dell'Italia et al., 1985). Inotropic therapy with dobutamine may be more effective in increasing cardiac output in some patients, and monitoring with serial echocardiograms may also be useful to detect RV overdistention (Dell'Italia et al., 1985). Maintenance of atrioventricular synchrony is also important in these patients to optimize RV filling (Kinch & Ryan, 1994). For patients with continued hemodynamic instability, IABP may be useful, particularly because elevated RV pressures and volumes increase wall stress and oxygen consumption and decrease right coronary perfusion pressure, exacerbating RV ischemia.

Reperfusion of the occluded coronary artery is also crucial. A study using direct angioplasty demonstrated that restoration of normal flow resulted in dramatic recovery of RV function and a mortality rate of only 2%, whereas unsuccessful reperfusion was associated with persistent hemodynamic compromise and a mortality of 58% (Bowers et al., 1998).

Cardiogenic Shock

EPIDEMIOLOGY AND PATHOPHYSIOLOGY

Cardiogenic shock, resulting either from LV pump failure or from mechanical complications, represents the leading cause of in-hospi-

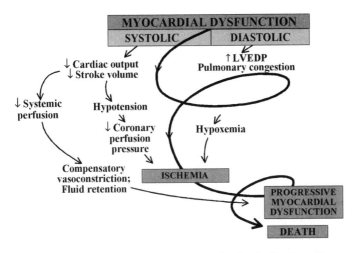

Fig. 4. The "downward spiral" in cardiogenic shock. Stroke volume and cardiac output fall with left ventricular (LV) dysfunction, producing hypotension and tachycardia that reduce coronary blood flow. Increasing ventricular diastolic pressure reduces coronary blood flow, and increased wall stress elevates myocardial oxygen requirements. All of these factors combine to worsen ischemia. The falling cardiac output also compromises systemic perfusion. Compensatory mechanisms include sympathetic stimulation and fluid retention to increase preload. These mechanisms can actually worsen cardiogenic shock by increasing myocardial oxygen demand and afterload. Thus, a vicious circle can be established. LVEDP, left ventricular end-diastolic pressure. (Adapted with permission from Hollenberg et al. 1999.)

tal death after MI (Hollenberg et al., 1999). Despite advances in management of heart failure and acute MI, until very recently, clinical outcomes in patients with cardiogenic shock have been poor, with reported mortality rates ranging from 50 to 80% (Goldberg et al., 1999). Patients may have cardiogenic shock at initial presentation, but shock often evolves over several hours (Hochman et al., 1995; Holmes et al., 1995).

Cardiac dysfunction in patients with cardiogenic shock is usually initiated by MI or ischemia. The myocardial dysfunction resulting from ischemia worsens that ischemia, creating a downward spiral (Fig. 4). Compensatory mechanisms that retain fluid in an attempt to maintain cardiac output may add to the vicious cycle and further increase diastolic filling pressures. The interruption of this cycle of myocardial dysfunction and ischemia forms the basis for the therapeutic regimens for cardiogenic shock.

INITIAL MANAGEMENT

Maintenance of adequate oxygenation and ventilation are critical. Many patients require intubation and mechanical ventilation, if only to reduce the work of breathing and facilitate sedation and stabilization before cardiac catheterization. Electrolyte abnormalities should be corrected, and morphine (or fentanyl if systolic pressure is compromised) used to relieve pain and anxiety, thus reducing excessive sympathetic activity and decreasing oxygen demand, preload, and afterload. Arrhythmias and heart block may have major effects on cardiac output, and should be corrected promptly with antiarrhythmic drugs, cardioversion, or pacing.

The initial approach to the hypotensive patient should include fluid resuscitation unless frank pulmonary edema is present. Patients are commonly diaphoretic and relative hypovolemia may be present in as many as 20% of patients with cardiogenic shock. Fluid infusion is best initiated with predetermined boluses titrated to clinical endpoints of heart rate, urine output, and blood pressure. Ischemia produces diastolic as well as systolic dysfunction, and thus elevated filling pressures may be necessary to maintain stroke volume in patients with cardiogenic shock. Patients who do not respond rapidly to initial fluid boluses or those with poor physiological reserve should be considered for invasive hemodynamic monitoring. Optimal filling pressures vary from patient to patient; hemodynamic monitoring can be used to construct a Starling curve at the bedside, identifying the filling pressure at which cardiac output is maximized. Maintenance of adequate preload is particularly important in patients with RV infarction.

When arterial pressure remains inadequate, therapy with vasopressor agents may be required to maintain coronary perfusion pressure. Maintenance of adequate blood pressure is essential to break the vicious cycle of progressive hypotension with further myocardial ischemia. Dopamine increases both blood pressure and cardiac output, and is usually the initial choice in patients with systolic pressures less than 80 mmHg. When hypotension remains refractory, norepinephrine may be necessary to maintain organ perfusion pressure. Phenylephrine, a selective α-1 adrenergic agonist, may be useful when tachyarrhythmias limit therapy with other vasopressors. Vasopressor infusions need to be titrated carefully in patients with cardiogenic shock to maximize coronary perfusion pressure with the least possible increase in myocardial oxygen demand. Hemodynamic monitoring, with serial measurements of cardiac output, filling pressures (and other parameters, such as mixed venous oxygen saturation), allows for titration of the dosage of vasoactive agents to the minimum dosage required to achieve the chosen therapeutic goals (Hollenberg & Hoyt, 1997).

Following initial stabilization and restoration of adequate blood pressure, tissue perfusion should be assessed. If tissue perfusion remains inadequate, inotropic support or IABP should be initiated. If tissue perfusion is adequate but significant pulmonary congestion remains, diuretics may be employed. Vasodilators can be considered as well, depending on the blood pressure.

In patients with inadequate tissue perfusion and adequate intravascular volume, cardiovascular support with inotropic agents should be initiated. Dobutamine, a selective β1-adrenergic receptor agonist, can improve myocardial contractility and increase cardiac output, and is the initial agent of choice in patients with systolic pressures greater than 80 mmHg. Dobutamine may exacerbate hypotension in some patients, and can precipitate tachyarrhythmias. Use of dopamine may be preferable if systolic pressure is less than 80 mmHg, although tachycardia and increased peripheral resistance may worsen myocardial ischemia. In some situations, a combination of dopamine and dobutamine can be more effective than either agent used alone. Phosphodiesterase inhibitors such as milrinone are less arrhythmogenic than catecholamines, but have the potential to cause hypotension, and should be used with caution in patients with tenuous clinical status.

IABP counterpulsation reduces systolic afterload and augments diastolic perfusion pressure, increasing cardiac output and improving coronary blood flow (Willerson et al., 1975). These beneficial effects, in contrast to those of inotropic or vasopressor agents, occur without an increase in oxygen demand. IABP does not, however, produce a significant improvement in blood flow distal to a critical coronary stenosis, and has not been shown to improve mortality when used alone without reperfusion therapy or revascularization.

In patients with cardiogenic shock and compromised tissue perfusion, IABP can be an essential support mechanism to stabilize patients and allow time for definitive therapeutic measures to be undertaken (Bates et al., 1998; Willerson et al., 1975). In appropriate settings, more intensive support with mechanical assist devices may also be implemented.

REPERFUSION THERAPY

Although thrombolytic therapy reduces the likelihood of subsequent development of shock after initial presentation (Holmes et al., 1995), its role in the management of patients who have already developed shock is less certain. The available randomized trials have not demonstrated that fibrinolytic therapy reduces mortality in patients with established cardiogenic shock. On the other hand, in the SHOCK Registry (Sanborn et al., 2000), patients treated with fibrinolytic therapy had a lower in-hospital mortality rate than those who were not (54 versus 64%, $p = 0.005$), even after adjustment for age and revascularization status (OR 0.70, $p = 0.027$).

Fibrinolytic therapy is clearly less effective in patients with cardiogenic shock than in those without. The explanation for this lack of efficacy appears to be the low reperfusion rate achieved in this subset of patients. The reasons for decreased thrombolytic efficacy in patients with cardiogenic probably include hemodynamic, mechanical, and metabolic factors that prevent achievement and maintenance of infarct-related artery patency (Becker, 1993). Attempts to increase reperfusion rates by increasing blood pressure with aggressive inotropic and pressor therapy and IABP counterpulsation make theoretic sense, and two small studies support the notion that vasopressor therapy to increase aortic pressure improves thrombolytic efficacy (Becker, 1993; Garber et al., 1995). The use of IABP to augment aortic diastolic pressure may increase the effectiveness of thrombolytics as well.

To date, emergency percutaneous revascularization is the only intervention that has been shown to consistently reduce mortality rates in patients with cardiogenic shock. An extensive body of observational and registry studies has shown consistent benefits from revascularization. Notable among these is the the GUSTO-1 trial, in which patients treated with an "aggressive" strategy (coronary angiography performed within 24 hours of shock onset with revascularization by PTCA or bypass surgery) had significantly lower mortality (38% compared with 62%) (Berger et al., 1997). The National Registry of Myocardial Infarction-2 (NRMI-2), collected 26,280 shock patients with cardiogenic shock in the setting of MI between 1994 and 1997, similarly supported the association between revascularization and survival (Rogers et al., 2000). Improved short-term mortality was noted in those who then underwent revascularization during the reference hospitalization, either via PTCA (12.8 mortality versus 43.9%) or CABG (6.5 versus 23.9%) (Rogers et al., 2000). These data complement the GUSTO-1 substudy data and are important, not only because of the sheer number of patients from whom these values are derived, but also because NRMI-2 was a national cross-sectional study that more closely represents general clinical practice than carefully selected trial populations. These studies cannot be regarded as definitive because of their retrospective design, but two randomized controlled trials have now evaluated revascularization for patients with MI.

The SHOCK study was a randomized, multicenter international trial that assigned patients with cardiogenic shock to receive optimal medical management—including IABP and thrombolytic therapy—or to cardiac catheterization with revascularization using PTCA or CABG (Hochman et al., 1999, 2001) The trial enrolled 302 patients and was powered to detect a 20% absolute decrease in 30-day all-cause mortality rates. Mortality at 30 days was 46.7% in patients treated with early intervention and 56% in patients treated with initial medical stabilization, but this difference did not quite reach statistical significance ($p = 0.11$) (Hochman et al., 1999). At 6 months, the absolute risk reduction with early invasive therapy in the SHOCK trial was 13% (50.3% compared with 63.1%, $p = 0.027$) (Hochman et al., 1999), and this risk reduction was maintained at 12 months (mortality 53.3 versus 66.4%, $p < 0.03$) (Hochman et al., 2001). Subgroup analysis showed a substantial improvement in mortality rates in patients younger than 75 years of age at both 30 days (41.4 versus 56.8%, $p = 0.01$) and 6 months (44.9 versus 65.0%, $p = 0.003$) (Hochman et al., 1999).

The SMASH trial was independently conceived and had a very similar design, although a more rigid definition of cardiogenic shock resulted in enrollment of sicker patients and a higher mortality (Urban et al., 1999). The trial was terminated early because of difficulties in patient recruitment, and enrolled only 55 patients. In the SMASH trial, a similar trend in 30-day absolute mortality reduction similar to that in the SHOCK trial of 9% was observed (69% mortality in the invasive group versus 78% in the medically managed group, RR = 0.88, 95% CI = 0.6–1.2, p = NS) (Urban et al., 1999). This benefit was also maintained at 1 year.

When the results of both the SHOCK and SMASH trials are put into perspective with results from other randomized, controlled trials of patients with acute MI, an important point emerges: despite the moderate relative risk reduction (for the SHOCK trial 0.72, CI 0.54–0.95, for the SMASH trial, 0.88, CI, 0.60–1.20) the absolute benefit is important, with 9 lives saved for 100 patients treated at 30 days in both trials, and 13.2 lives saved for 100 patients treated at 1 year in the SHOCK trial. This latter figure corresponds to a number needed to treat of 7.6, one of the lowest figures ever observed in a randomized, controlled trial of cardiovascular disease.

On the basis of these randomized trials, the presence of cardiogenic shock in the setting of acute MI is a class I indication for emergency revascularization, either by PCI or CABG (Ryan et al., 1999).

REFERENCES

1. Ambrose JA, Martinez EE. A new paradigm for plaque stabilization. Circulation 105:2000–2004, 2002.
2. Andersen HR, Nielsen TT, Rasmussen K, et al. A comparison of coronary angioplasty with fibrinolytic therapy in acute myocardial infarction. N Engl J Med 349:733–742, 2003.
3. Antman EM, Cohen M, Radley D, et al. Assessment of the treatment effect of enoxaparin for unstable angina/non-Q-wave myocardial infarction. TIMI 11B–ESSENCE meta-analysis. Circulation 100:1602–1608, 1999.
4. Assessment of the Safety and Efficacy of a New Thrombolytic Investigators. Single-bolus tenecteplase compared with front-loaded alteplase in acute myocardial infarction: the ASSENT-2 double-blind randomised trial. Lancet 354: 716–722, 1999.
5. Aversano T, Aversano LT, Passamani E, et al. Thrombolytic therapy vs primary percutaneous coronary intervention for myocardial infarction in patients presenting to hospitals without on-site cardiac surgery: a randomized controlled trial. JAMA 287:1943–1951, 2002.
6. Bates ER, Stomel RJ, Hochman JS, Ohman EM. The use of intraaortic balloon counterpulsation as an adjunct to reperfusion therapy in cardiogenic shock. Int J Cardiol 65 Suppl 1:S37–42, 1998.
7. Becker RC. Hemodynamic, mechanical, and metabolic determinants of thrombolytic efficacy: a theoretic framework for assessing the limitations of

thrombolysis in patients with cardiogenic shock. Am Heart J 125:919–929, 1993.

8. Berger PB, Holmes DR, Jr., Stebbins AL, Bates ER, Califf RM, Topol EJ. Impact of an aggressive invasive catheterization and revascularization strategy on mortality in patients with cardiogenic shock in the Global Utilization of Streptokinase and Tissue Plasminogen Activator for Occluded Coronary Arteries (GUSTO-I) trial. An observational study. Circulation 96:122–127, 1997.

9. Boden WE, O'Rourke RA, Crawford MH, et al., and Veterans Affairs Non-Q-Wave Infarction Strategies in Hospital (VANQWISH) Trial Investigators. Outcomes in patients with acute non-Q-wave myocardial infarction randomly assigned to an invasive as compared with a conservative management strategy. N Engl J Med 338:1785–1792, 1998.

10. Bolooki H. Emergency cardiac procedures in patients in cardiogenic shock due to complications of coronary artery disease. Circulation 79:I137–I148, 1989.

11. Bowers TR, O'Neill WW, Grines C, Pica MC, Safian RD, Goldstein JA. Effect of reperfusion on biventricular function and survival after right ventricular infarction. N Engl J Med 338:933–940, 1998.

12. Braunwald E. Unstable angina. A classification. Circulation 80:410–414, 1989.

13. Cairns JA, Gent M, Singer J, et al. Aspirin, sulfinpyrazone, or both in unstable angina. Results of a Canadian multicenter trial. N Engl J Med 313:1369–1375, 1985.

14. Cannon CP, Gibson CM, Lambrew CT, et al. Relationship of symptom-onset-to-balloon time and door-to-balloon time with mortality in patients undergoing angioplasty for acute myocardial infarction. JAMA 283:2941–2947, 2000.

15. Cannon CP, Weintraub WS, Demopoulos LA, et al. Comparison of early invasive and conservative strategies in patients with unstable coronary syndromes treated with the glycoprotein IIb/IIIa inhibitor tirofiban. N Engl J Med 344:1879–1887, 2001.

16. Canto JG, Every NR, Magid DJ, et al. The volume of primary angioplasty procedures and survival after acute myocardial infarction. National Registry of Myocardial Infarction 2 Investigators. N Engl J Med 342:1573–1580, 2000.

17. CAPRIE Steering Committee. A randomised, blinded, trial of clopidogrel versus aspirin in patients at risk of ischaemic events (CAPRIE). Lancet 348:1329–1339, 1996.

18. CAPTURE Investigators. Randomised placebo-controlled trial of abciximab before and during coronary intervention in refractory unstable angina: the CAPTURE Study. Lancet 349:1429–1435, 1997.

19. Chew DP Moliterno DJ. A critical appraisal of platelet glycoprotein IIb/IIIa inhibition. J Am Coll Cardiol 36:2028–2035. 2000.

20. Croft CH, Nicod P, Corbett JR, et al. Detection of acute right ventricular infarction by right precordial electrocardiography. Am J Cardiol 50:421–427, 1982.

21. Dargie HJ. Effect of carvedilol on outcome after myocardial infarction in patients with left-ventricular dysfunction: the CAPRICORN randomised trial. Lancet 357:1385–1390, 2001.

22. Dell'Italia LJ, Starling MR, Blumhardt R, Lasher JC, O'Rourke RA. Comparative effects of volume loading, dobutamine, and nitroprusside in patients with predominant right ventricular infarction. Circulation 72:1327–1335, 1985.

23. Edner M, Bonarjee VV, Nilsen DW, Berning J, Carstensen S, Caidahl K. Effect of enalapril initiated early after acute myocardial infarction on heart failure parameters, with reference to clinical class and echocardiographic determinants. CONSENSUS II Multi-Echo Study Group. Clin Cardiol 19:543–548, 1996.

24. Ellis SG, da Silva ER, Heyndrickx G, et al., and Investigators. R. Randomized comparison of rescue angioplasty with conservative management of patients with early failure of thrombolysis for acute anterior myocardial infarction. Circulation 90:2280–2284, 1994.

25. Ferguson JJ, Califf RM, Antman EM, et al. Enoxaparin vs unfractionated heparin in high-risk patients with non-ST-segment elevation acute coronary syndromes managed with an intended early invasive strategy: primary results of the SYNERGY randomized trial. JAMA 292:45–54, 2004.

26. First International Study of Infarct Survival Collaborative Group. Randomised trial of intravenous atenolol among 16 027 cases of suspected acute myocardial infarction: ISIS-1. Lancet 2:57–66, 1986.

27. FRagmin and Fast Revascularisation During InStability in Coronary Artery Disease Investigators. Invasive compared with non-invasive treatment in unstable coronary- artery disease: FRISC II prospective randomised multicentre study. Lancet 354:708–715, 1999.

28. Frick MH, Elo O, Haapa K, et al. Helsinki heart study: primary-prevention trial with gemfibrozil in middle-aged men with dyslipidemia. Safety of treatment, changes in risk factors, and incidence of coronary heart disease. New Engl J Med 317:1237–1245, 1987.

29. Garber PJ, Mathieson AL, Ducas J, Patton JN, Geddes JS, Prewitt RM. Thrombolytic therapy in cardiogenic shock: effect of increased aortic pressure and rapid tPA administration. Can J Cardiol 11:30–36, 1995.

30. Gibbons RJ, Abrams J, Chatterjee K, et al. ACC/AHA 2002 guideline update for the management of patients with chronic stable angina—summary article: a report of the American College of Cardiology/American Heart Association Task Force on Practice Guidelines (Committee on the Management of Patients With Chronic Stable Angina). Circulation 107:149–158, 2003.

31. Gibson RS, Boden WE, Theroux P, et al. Diltiazem and reinfarction in patients with non-Q-wave myocardial infarction. Results of a double-blind, randomized, multicenter trial. N Engl J Med 315:423–429, 1986.

32. Global Use of Strategies to Open Occluded Coronary Arteries (GUSTO III) Investigators. A comparison of reteplase with alteplase for acute myocardial infarction. N Engl J Med 337:1118–1123, 1997.

33. Goldberg RJ, Samad NA, Yarzebski J, Gurwitz J, Bigelow C, Gore JM. Temporal trends in cardiogenic shock complicating acute myocardial infarction. N Engl J Med 340:1162–1168, 1999.

34. Grines C, Patel A, Zijlstra F, Weaver WD, Granger C, Simes RJ. Primary coronary angioplasty compared with intravenous thrombolytic therapy for acute myocardial infarction: six-month follow up and analysis of individual patient data from randomized trials. Am Heart J 145:47–57, 2003.

35. Grines CL, Browne KF, Marco J, et al. A comparison of immediate angioplasty with thrombolytic therapy for acute myocardial infarction. The Primary

Angioplasty in Myocardial Infarction Study Group. N Engl J Med 328:673–679, 1993.

36. Gruppo Italiano per lo Studio della Sopravvinza nell'Infarto Miocardico (GISSI). GISSI-3: effects of lisinopril and transdermal glyceryl trinitrate singly and together on 6-week mortality and ventricular function after acute myocardial infarction. Lancet 343:1115–1122, 1994.

37. Gruppo Italiano per lo Studio della Streptochinasi nell'Infarto Miocardico (GISSI). Effectiveness of intravenous thrombolytic treatment in acute myocardial infarction. Lancet 1:397–402, 1986.

38. GUSTO Angiographic Investigators. The effects of tissue plasminogen activator, streptokinase, or both on coronary-artery patency, ventricular function, and survival after acute myocardial infarction. N Engl J Med 329:1615–1622, 1993.

39. GUSTO IIb Investigators. A comparison of recombinant hirudin with heparin for the treatment of acute coronary syndromes. N Engl J Med 335:775–782, 1996.

40. GUSTO Investigators. An international randomized trial comparing four thrombolytic strategies for acute myocardial infarction. New Engl J Med 329: 673–682, 1993.

41. Hochman JS, Boland J, Sleeper LA, et al. and Investigators SR. Current spectrum of cardiogenic shock and effect of early revascularization on mortality. Results of an International Registry. Circulation 91:873–881, 1995.

42. Hochman JS, Sleeper LA, Webb JG, et al. and SHOCK (Should We Emergently Revascularize Occluded Coronaries for Cardiogenic Shock) Investigators. Early revascularization in acute myocardial infarction complicated by cardiogenic shock. N Engl J Med 341:625–634, 1999.

43. Hochman JS, Sleeper LA, White HD, et al. One-year survival following early revascularization for cardiogenic shock. JAMA 285:190–192. 2001.

44. Hollenberg SM Hoyt JW. Pulmonary artery catheters in cardiovascular disease. New Horizons 5:207–213, 1997.

45. Hollenberg SM, Kavinsky CJ, Parrillo JE. Cardiogenic shock. Ann Intern Med 131:47–59, 1999.

46. Holmes DR, Jr., Bates ER, Kleiman NS, et al. Contemporary reperfusion therapy for cardiogenic shock: the GUSTO-I trial experience. The GUSTO-I Investigators. Global Utilization of Streptokinase and Tissue Plasminogen Activator for Occluded Coronary Arteries. J Am Coll Cardiol 26:668–674, 1995.

47. ISIS-2 (Second International Study of Infarct Survival) Collaborative Group. Randomised trial of intravenous streptokinase, oral aspirin, both, or neither among 17,187 cases of suspected acute myocardial infarction: ISIS-2. Lancet 2:349–360, 1988.

48. ISIS-4 (Fourth International Study of Infarct Survival) Study Group. ISIS-4: a randomised factorial trial assessing early oral captopril, oral mononitrate, and intravenous magnesium sulphate in 58,050 patients with suspected acute myocardial infarction. Lancet 345:669–685, 1995.

49. Jaffe AS, Ravkilde J, Roberts R, et al. It's time for a change to a troponin standard. Circulation 102:1216–1220, 2000.

50. Katus HA, Remppis A, Neumann FJ, et al. Diagnostic efficiency of troponin T measurements in acute myocardial infarction. Circulation 83:902–912, 1991.

51. Keeley EC, Boura JA, Grines CL. Primary angioplasty versus intravenous thrombolytic therapy for acute myocardial infarction: a quantitative review of 23 randomised trials. Lancet 361:13–20, 2003.

52. Khan SS Gray RJ. Valvular emergencies. Cardiol Clin 9:689–709, 1991.

53. Killen DA, Piehler JM, Borkon AM, Gorton ME, Reed WA. Early repair of postinfarction ventricular septal rupture. Ann Thorac Surg 63:138–142, 1997.

54. Kinch JW Ryan TJ. Right ventricular infarction. N Engl J Med 330:1211–1217, 1994.

55. Lauler DP. Magnesium—coming of age. Am J Cardiol 63:1g–3g, 1989.

56. Lee TH Goldman L. Serum enzyme assays in the diagnosis of acute myocardial infarction. Recommendations based on a quantitative analysis. Ann Intern Med 105:221–233, 1986.

57. Lewis HD, Jr., Davis JW, Archibald DG, et al. Protective effects of aspirin against acute myocardial infarction and death in men with unstable angina. Results of a Veterans Administration Cooperative Study. N Engl J Med 309:396–403, 1983.

58. Libby P. Current concepts of the pathogenesis of the acute coronary syndromes. Circulation 104:365–372. 2001.

59. Lipid Research Clinics Program. The lipid research clinics coronary primary prevention trial results. II. The relationship of reduction in incidence of coronary heart disease to cholesterol lowering. JAMA 251:365–374, 1984.

60. Long-Term Intervention with Pravastatin in Ischaemic Disease (LIPID) Study Group. Prevention of cardiovascular events and death with pravastatin in patients with coronary heart disease and a broad range of initial cholesterol levels. N Engl J Med 339:1349–1357, 1998.

61. MacMahon S, Collins R, Peto R, Koster RW, Yusuf S. Effects of prophylactic lidocaine in suspected acute myocardial infarction. An overview of results from the randomized, controlled trials. Jama 260:1910–1916, 1988.

62. MIAMI Trial Research Group. Metoprolol in acute myocardial infarction (MIAMI). A randomised placebo-controlled international trial. Eur Heart J 6:199–226, 1985.

63. Ohman EM, Armstrong PW, Christenson RH, et al. and Investigators GI. Cardiac troponin T levels for risk stratification in acute myocardial ischemia. New Engl J Med 335:133–1341, 1996.

64. Oler A, Whooley MA, Oler J, Grady D. Adding heparin to aspirin reduces the incidence of myocardial infarction and death in patients with unstable angina. A meta-analysis. Jama 276:811–815, 1996.

65. PARAGON Investigators. International, randomized, controlled trial of lamifiban (a platelet glycoprotein IIb/IIIa inhibitor), heparin, or both in unstable angina. Circulation 97:2386–2395, 1998.

66. Pfeffer MA, Braunwald E, Moye LA, et al. and Investigators. S. Effect of captopril on mortality and morbidity in patients with left ventricular dysfunction after myocardial infarction. Results of the Survival and Ventricular Enlargement Trial. N Engl J Med 327:669–677, 1992.

67. Platelet Receptor Inhibition in Ischemic Syndrome Management (PRISM) Study Investigators. A Comparison of Aspirin plus Tirofiban with Aspirin plus Heparin for Unstable Angina. N Engl J Med 338:1498–1505, 1998.

68. Platelet Receptor Inhibition in Ischemic Syndrome Management in Patients Limited by Unstable Signs and Symptoms (PRISM-PLUS) Study Investigators. Inhibition of the platelet glycoprotein IIb/IIIa receptor with tirofiban in unstable angina and non-Q-wave myocardial infarction. N Engl J Med 338: 1488–1497, 1998.

69. Rapaport E. Serum enzymes and isoenzymes in the diagnosis of acute myocardial infarction. Part II: Isoenzymes. Mod Concepts Cardiovasc Dis 46:47–50, 1977.

70. Reardon MJ, Carr CL, Diamond A, et al. Ischemic left ventricular free wall rupture: prediction, diagnosis, and treatment. Ann Thorac Surg 64:1509–1513, 1997.

71. Rogers WJ, Canto JG, Lambrew CT, et al. Temporal trends in the treatment of over 1.5 million patients with myocardial infarction in the US from 1990 through 1999: the National Registry of Myocardial Infarction 1, 2 and 3. J Am Coll Cardiol 36:2056–2063, 2000.

72. Ryan TJ, Antman EM, Brooks NH, et al. 1999 update: ACC/AHA guidelines for the management of patients with acute myocardial infarction. A report of the American College of Cardiology/American Heart Association Task Force on Practice Guidelines (Committee on Management of Acute Myocardial Infarction). J Am Coll Cardiol 34:890–911. 1999.

73. Sacks FM, Pfeffer MA, Moye LA, et al. The effect of pravastatin on coronary events after myocardial infarction in patients with average cholesterol levels. New Engl J Med 335:1001–1009, 1996.

74. Sanborn TA, Sleeper LA, Bates ER, et al. Impact of thrombolysis, intra-aortic balloon pump counterpulsation, and their combination in cardiogenic shock complicating acute myocardial infarction: a report from the SHOCK Trial Registry. SHould we emergently revascularize Occluded Coronaries for cardiogenic shocK? J Am Coll Cardiol 36:1123–1129. 2000.

75. Scandinavian Simvastatin Survival Study Group. Randomised trial of cholesterol lowering in 4444 patients with coronary heart disease: the Scandinavian Simvastatin Survival Study (4S). Lancet 344:1383–1389, 1994.

76. Simoons ML. Effect of glycoprotein IIb/IIIa receptor blocker abciximab on outcome in patients with acute coronary syndromes without early coronary revascularisation: the GUSTO IV-ACS randomised trial. Lancet 357:1915–1924, 2001.

77. Spodick DH. Diagnostic electrocardiographic sequences in acute pericarditis. Significance of PR segment and PR vector changes. Circulation 48:575–580, 1973.

78. The International Collaborative Study Group. Reduction of infarct size with the early use of timolol in acute myocardial infarction. New Engl J Med 310:9–15, 1984.

79. The PURSUIT Trial Investigators. Inhibition of platelet glycoprotein IIb/IIIa with eptifibatide in patients with acute coronary syndromes. N Engl J Med 339: 436–443, 1998.

80. Theroux P, Ouimet H, McCans J, et al. Aspirin, heparin, or both to treat acute unstable angina. N Engl J Med 319:1105–1111, 1988.

81. TIMI Investigators. Effects of tissue plasminogen activator and a comparison of early invasive and conservative strategies in unstable angina and non-Q-

wave myocardial infarction. Results of the TIMI IIIB Trial. Circulation 89: 1545–1556, 1994.

82. TIMI Study Group. Comparison of invasive and conservative strategies after treatment with intravenous tissue plasminogen activator in acute myocardial infarction. Results of the thrombolysis in myocardial infarction (TIMI) phase II trial. N Engl J Med 320:618–627, 1989.

83. TIMI Study Group. The Thrombolysis in Myocardial Infarction (TIMI) trial. Phase I findings. N Engl J Med 312:932–936, 1985.

84. Urban P, Stauffer JC, Bleed D, et al. A randomized evaluation of early revascularization to treat shock complicating acute myocardial infarction. The (Swiss) Multicenter Trial of Angioplasty for Shock-(S)MASH. Eur Heart J 20: 1030–1038, 1999.

85. Widimsky P, Budesinsky T, Vorac D, et al. Long distance transport for primary angioplasty vs immediate thrombolysis in acute myocardial infarction. Final results of the randomized national multicentre trial—PRAGUE-2. Eur Heart J 24:94–104, 2003.

86. Willerson JT, Curry GC, Watson JT, et al. Intraaortic balloon counterpulsation in patients in cardiogenic shock, medically refractory left ventricular failure and/or recurrent ventricular tachycardia. Am J Med 58:183–191, 1975.

87. Yusuf S, Zhao F, Mehta SR, Chrolavicius S, Tognoni G, Fox KK. Effects of clopidogrel in addition to aspirin in patients with acute coronary syndromes without ST-segment elevation. N Engl J Med 345:494–502, 2001.

88. Zehender M, Kasper W, Kauder E, et al. Right ventricular infarction as an independent predictor of prognosis after acute inferior myocardial infarction. New Engl J Med 328:981–988, 1993.

2   Arrhythmias

INTRODUCTION

The physiological impact of an arrhythmia depends on ventricular response rate, duration of arrhythmia, and underlying cardiac function. Bradyarrhythmias may decrease cardiac output owing to heart rate alone in patients with a relatively fixed stroke volume. Loss of atrial contraction may cause a dramatic increase in pulmonary artery pressures in patients with hypertension and diastolic dysfunction. Similarly, tachyarrhythmias can decrease diastolic filling time and reduce cardiac output, resulting in hypotension and possible myocardial ischemia. The impact of a given arrhythmia depends on the patient's cardiac physiology and function. Treatment is determined by the hemodynamic insult. In this chapter, a systematic approach to diagnosis and evaluation of predisposing factors is presented, followed by consideration of specific arrhythmias.

ARRHYTHMIA DIAGNOSIS
Basic Principles

The first principle in managing arrhythmias is to appropriately treat the patient, not the electrocardiogram (ECG). Accordingly, one must first decide whether the observed arrhythmia may be an artifact. If the arrhythmia is real and sustained, it must be determined whether is has important clinical consequences.

The next step is to establish the urgency of treatment. Clinical assessment includes evaluation of pulse, blood pressure, peripheral perfusion, and consideration of myocardial ischemia and/or congestive heart failure. If the patient loses consciousness or becomes hemodynamically unstable in the presence of a tachyarrhythmia

From: *Current Clinical Practice: Cardiology in Family Practice:*
A Practical Guide
By: S. M. Hollenberg and T. Walker © Humana Press Inc., Totowa, NJ

other than sinus tachycardia, prompt cardioversion may be indicated regardless of anticoagulation status. If the patient is stable, there is often time to establish the rhythm diagnosis and decide upon the most appropriate treatment. Bradyarrhythmias produce less of a diagnostic challenge and treatment options are relatively straight-forward.

The goals of antiarrhythmic therapy depend on the type of rhythm disturbance. The initial goal for the treatment of an arrhythmia is to stabilize the hemodynamics and ventricular response. The next goal is to restore sinus rhythm if possible. If restoration of sinus rhythm cannot be achieved, prevention of complications is important.

Classification of Arrhythmias

Arrhythmias are usually classified according to anatomic origin, either supraventricular or ventricular. The most common supraventricular arrhythmia is sinus tachycardia, followed by atrial fibrillation, ectopic atrial or junctional tachycardia, multifocal atrial tachycardia, atrioventricular (AV) nodal reentry tachycardias, and accessory pathway tachycardias. Ventricular arrhythmias are most commonly premature ventricular beats, ventricular tachycardia, and ventricular fibrillation.

It is sometimes useful to consider tachyarrhythmias from a treatment standpoint. Tachyarrhythmias that traverse the AV node can often be controlled by pharmacologically altering AV nodal conduction. Rhythms that traverse the AV node include atrial fibrillation and flutter, ectopic atrial and junctional tachycardias, multifocal atrial tachycardia, and AV nodal reentry tachycardias. Rhythms that do not utilize the AV node include accessory pathway tachycardias through a bypass tract, ventricular tachycardia, and ventricular fibrillation. When the arrhythmia does not utilize the AV node, slowing AV nodal conduction can be dangerous.

Rhythm Diagnosis

A comprehensive description of the diagnosis of arrhythmias is beyond the scope of this manuscript. A 12-lead ECG with a long rhythm strip and a previously obtained 12-lead ECG for comparison are ideal; If a previous ECG is not available, a systematic approach using a current 12-lead ECG is essential. An approach is outlined using the following five steps (Marriott, 1988).

1. LOCATE THE P-WAVE

P-waves are often best seen in leads II and V_1. Normal P-waves are upright in leads II, III, and aVF, and may be biphasic in leads II and V_1. If P-waves are present and always followed by a QRS complex, the rhythm is most likely sinus tachycardia, which usually occurs at a rate between 100 and 180 in adults. Ectopic atrial and junctional tachycardias often present with negative P-waves in leads II, III, and aVF. If P-waves are present and the rhythm is irregular, the rhythm is most likely atrial fibrillation. If the P-wave is buried in the QRS or ST segment, the rhythm is most likely AV nodal reentry tachycardia, which usually present with atrial rates from 140 to 220. If there are multiple P-waves followed by a single QRS, especially if the atrial rate is near 300, the rhythm is most likely atrial flutter. If no P-waves are present, the rhythm is most likely atrial fibrillation.

2. ESTABLISH THE RELATIONSHIP BETWEEN THE P-WAVE AND QRS

If there are more P-waves than QRS complexes, then AV block is present. If there are more QRS complexes than P-waves, the rhythm is likely an accelerated junctional or ventricular rhythm. If the relationship of the P-wave and QRS is 1:1, then measurement of the PR interval can yield useful diagnostic clues.

3. EXAMINE THE QRS MORPHOLOGY

A narrow QRS complex (<0.12 ms) indicates a supraventricular arrhythmia. A wide QRS complex can be either ventricular tachycardia or supraventricular tachycardia with either a pre-existing bundle branch block, or, less commonly, aberrant ventricular conduction or an antegrade accessory pathway.

4. SEARCH FOR OTHER CLUES

The clues to guide appropriate therapy depend on the situation. Carotid sinus massage increases AV block and can either break a supraventricular tachycardia or bring out previously undetected flutter waves. Any patient with a ventricular rate of exactly 150 beats per minute (bpm) should be suspected of having atrial flutter with 2:1 AV block. A rate greater than 200 bpm in an otherwise healthy adult should raise the suspicion of an accessory pathway. Severe left axis deviation (–60° to 120°) during tachycardia suggests a ventricular origin, as does AV dissociation, fusion beats (which result from simultaneous activation of two foci, one ventricular and one supraventricular), and capture beats (beats that capture the ventricles and are conducted with a narrow complex, ruling out fixed bundle branch block). Grouped beating or more P-waves than QRS complexes suggests the possibility of second-degree AV block.

ATRIAL FIBRILLATION
Etiology and Pathophysiology

Atrial fibrillation is the most common sustained tachycardia encountered in clinical practice. It is estimated that 2.2 million Americans have paroxysmal or persistent atrial fibrillation. The prevalence increases with age and is more common in men than women (Go et al., 2001). The prevalence is 3.8% for persons greater than 60 years old and 9.0% for persons over 80 years old (Go et al., 2001).

Atrial fibrillation is characterized by uncoordinated atrial activity with an irregular ventricular response, usually rapid. Atrial fibrillation can occur with or without underlying structural heart disease or may be secondary to other predisposing conditions. Cardiac diseases associated with atrial fibrillation include hypertension, valvular heart disease, coronary artery disease (CAD), and cardiomyopathies. Atrial fibrillation has also been linked to alcohol ingestion, pulmonary embolism, hyperthyroidism, obstructive sleep apnea, chronic obstructive pulmonary disease , and is common following cardiac or thoracic surgery. Atrial fibrillation following an acute myocardial infarction (MI) carries a poor prognostic sign (Rathore et al., 2000).

Atrial fibrillation has been classified as paroxysmal, persistent, permanent, and lone (Fuster et al., 2001). Two or more episodes of atrial fibrillation has been defined as recurrent atrial fibrillation. Recurrent atrial fibrillation is further classified as either paroxysmal (terminates spontaneously) or persistent (sustained and does not convert to sinus rhythm without either pharmacological or electrical cardioversion). Permanent atrial fibrillation refers to long-standing atrial fibrillation (more than 1 year) in which cardioversion has not been indicated or attempted (Fuster et al., 2001). Lone atrial fibrillation refers to patients without structural heart disease or conditions predisposing to atrial fibrillation.

The mechanism of atrial fibrillation is not entirely clear. The conventional viewpoint was that multiple reentrant impulses wandering throughout the atria created continuous electrical activity, the multiple wavelet hypothesis (Jalife, 2003). More recently, focal origin from electrically active tissue situated in the pulmonary veins have been identified (Haissaguerre et al., 1998). Other foci include the right atrium, superior vena cava, and coronary sinus (Chen et al., 1999; Haissaguerre et al., 1998; Jais et al., 1997). The distinction between these mechanisms is more than merely academic because origin from discrete foci presents the possibility of treatment either by ablating these foci or isolating them from the rest of the atrium.

Atrial fibrillation results in loss of effective atrial contraction and AV synchrony. The variation in the RR interval leads to changing diastolic filling intervals and therefore varying stroke volumes of AV synchrony may have an adverse impact on cardiac output.

Clinical Features

The symptoms of atrial fibrillation result from the rapidity and irregularity of the ventricular response and the loss of AV synchrony. The most common symptoms include palpitations, dyspnea, fatigue, lightheadedness, chest pain, and syncope. However, some patients with atrial fibrillation are completely asymptomatic.

The initial workup should include a complete history and physical exam, ECG, thyroid function tests, chest radiograph, complete blood count, serum electrolytes, and transthoracic echocardiogram. The history should focus on the onset, duration, frequency, symptoms, precipitating or reversible factors, and terminating events of each episode.

The ECG shows absent P-waves and an irregularly irregular rhythm. Fibrillatory waves may be seen in the inferior leads, at a rate of 300–700 bpm. The ventricular rate is usually between 100 and 180 bpm, but may be slower if there is AV nodal conduction disease, high vagal tone, or drugs affecting AV nodal conduction. The ventricular rate may be regular if the patient is ventricular-paced or there is an AV block. A chest x-ray is useful to evaluate the lungs, cardiac silhouette, and pulmonary vasculature.

All patients with new-onset atrial fibrillation should be evaluated by echocardiography. Echocardiography should be performed to evaluate the left and right atrial size, left and right ventricular size and function, valvular abnormalities, or pericardial disease. Transthoracic echocardiography can occasionally detect left atrial thrombus but the sensitivity is low. Transesophageal echocardiography (TEE) is the most sensitive and specific technique for diagnosing a thrombus in the left atrium, and should be considered before cardioversion or after a suspected embolic event.

Exercise testing should be performed on patients with suspected ischemic heart disease and those being considered for type Ic antiarrhythmic drug therapy (Fuster et al., 2001). Holter or event monitors may be used to capture the arrhythmia in patients with paroxysmal atrial fibrillation and to evaluate rate control.

Therapy

The three goals of therapy for atrial fibrillation are to control the rate, to restore and maintain normal sinus rhythm, and to prevent complications. Recent clinical trials have created controversy concerning whether rhythm control is superior to rate control. The Atrial Fibrillation Follow-Up Investigation of Rhythm Management (AF-FIRM) study enrolled 4060 patients older than 65 with at least one risk factor for stroke or death in a randomized, controlled trial comparing a rhythm control strategy to rate control (Wyse et al., 2002). Patients were randomized to antiarrhythmic drugs or cardioversion to restore sinus rhythm, or AV nodal blocking agents. The rate-control groups were anticoagulated indefinitely. The rhythm-control groups were anticoagulated, but at the discretion of their physician could be stopped if they were in normal sinus rhythm for longer than 4 weeks. The composite endpoint (death, disabling stroke, disabling anoxic encephalopathy, major bleeding, cardiac arrest) was not statistically different, but overall mortality was higher in the rhythm-control group, although this was not statistically significant. The rhythm-control group had more hospitalization, and in a 5-year follow-up only 63% was in normal sinus rhythm. Stroke rates averaged 1% per year in both groups, and occurred mostly in patients who stopped taking warfarin or who were subtherapeutic (Wyse et al., 2002).

The Rate Control versus Electrical Cardioversion for Persistent Atrial Fibrillation (RACE) study was a similar randomized, controlled trial comparing rhythm versus rate control in 522 patients with persistent atrial fibrillation, 90% of whom had risk factors for stroke (Van Gelder et al., 2002). Patients in the rate-control group received β-blockers, calcium channel blockers (CCBs), or digoxin, and those in the rhythm group were cardioverted and maintained on sotalol. All patients received anticoagulation, but this could be discontinued in the rhythm-control group if sinus rhythm was achieved. There was no statistically significance in the composite endpoint (cardiovascular mortality, heart failure, thromboembolic events, bleeding, pacemaker implantation, drug side effects) in the rate-control (17.2%) and rhythm-control (22.6%) groups (Van Gelder et al., 2002). As with the AFFIRM trial, there were increased thromboembolic complications in the rhythm group, mainly among patients who discontinued anticoagulation therapy.

The Pharmacological Intervention in Atrial Fibrillation study was a rate versus rhythm trial enrolling 252 patients with persistent symptomatic atrial fibrillation, with symptomatic improvement as the primary endpoint (Hohnloser et al., 2000). The rate-control group was given diltiazem, whereas the rhythm group was given amiodarone; all patients were anticoagulated. Quality of life and symptoms improved in both groups to the same extent. The rhythm group had better exercise tolerance. More patients in the rhythm-control group were hospitalized and they suffered more drug side effects.

The Strategies of Treatment of Atrial Fibrillation pilot study examined the effects of rate versus rhythm control on death, cardiovascular events, cardiopulmonary resuscitation, or systemic emboli (Carlsson et al., 2003). The rate-control group received an AV nodal blocking medication (β-blocker, CCB, digoxin). The rhythm-control group received amiodarone or some other class I antiarrhythmic, or electrical cardioversion. Both groups were anticoagulated. There was no statistically significant difference in either the primary endpoint or the secondary endpoints (syncope, bleeding, worsening heart failure, quality of life). The rhythm-control group required more frequent hospitalizations with longer lengths of stay. At a 3-year follow-up, only 23% of the rhythm-control group was in sinus rhythm (Carlsson et al., 2003).

Based on these trials, either a rate-control or a rhythm-control strategy can be chosen, individualized to a particular patient. The initial priority in a patient presenting with atrial fibrillation is to control the ventricular rate acutely. This can be accomplished with either β-blockers or CCBs. If very rapid control is required, intravenous β-blockade with metoprolol (5 mg intravenously every 5 minutes up to three doses) or esmolol (500 µg/kg bolus and 50 µg/kg per minute infusion titrated up in 50 µg/kg per minute increments every 3 to 5 minutes up to 200 µg/kg per minute), followed by oral therapy can be used. Risks include hypotension, bronchospasm, and negative inotropic effects. Intravenous calcium channel blockade with diltiazem (10–20 mg intravenously over 2 minutes and then at 5–20 mg per hour intravenously) or verapamil (2.5 mg intravenously over 2 minutes, repeated every 15 minutes up to 15 mg), followed by oral therapy is equally acceptable. Risks include hypotension and heart failure. Digoxin is a second-line alternative that is much better for chronic than acute rate control, and is recommended in patients with heart failure (Snow et al., 2003). Digoxin can be loaded intravenously (1 mg load, usually 0.25 mg intravenously every 6 hours but can be given as 0.5 mg once followed by 0.25 mg every 3 hours for two doses) if necessary. Measurement of levels should be done at steady-state, and is not especially helpful in atrial fibrillation except in patients with suspected toxicity. Maintenance doses range from 0.125 to 0.375 mg per day, and require adjustment for renal insufficiency.

Chronically, rate control is needed to avoid the symptoms and hemodynamic instability caused by a rapid ventricular response. β-Blockers (atenolol, metoprolol, propranolol, esmolol), nondihydropyridine calcium antagonists (verapamil, diltiazem), and digoxin slow AV nodal conduction and are the recommended pharmacological agents for rate control. The current American College of Cardiology/American Heart Association/European Society of Cardiology (ACC/AHA/ESC) guidelines recommend dose titration to a resting heart rate of 60–80 and 90–115 bpm during exercise (Fuster et al., 2001). Digoxin provides rate control at rest but not with exercise, and is used in combination with β-blockers or CCBs or alone when they are not tolerated.

Hemodynamically unstable patients require emergent cardioversion, and those with acute heart failure or angina should be considered for urgent cardioversion. Electrical cardioversion may be more effective when the defibrillator pads are placed in an anterior–posterior orientation to direct the current through the atria.

Rhythm control is achieved either through synchronized external cardioversion or pharmacological cardioversion. The risk of thromboembolism is the same for electrical and pharmacological cardioversion. If the duration of atrial fibrillation less than 48 hours and the patient is at low thromboembolic risk, the patient should be heparinized, cardioverted, and given aspirin for 1 month. A patient at high risk (mitral valve disease, previous thromboembolism, severe left ventricular [LV] dysfunction) should be anticoagulated for 1 month before elective cardioversion. For patients presenting in atrial fibrillation for more than 48 hours or of unknown duration, intravenous heparin and oral warfarin should be initiated upon presentation. TEE can be used to evaluate for left atrial thrombus. If no thrombus is visualized, the patient can be safely cardioverted and then anticoagulated for 1 month (Manning et al., 1993) because recovery of atrial mechanical function may be delayed despite restoration of sinus rhythm. If a thrombus is seen, the patient should be anticoagulated for at least 3–4 weeks prior to elective cardioversion.

The use of pharmacological cardioversion should be based on the duration of the atrial fibrillation, presence or absence of structural heart disease, and persistent symptoms on rate-control agents. Before instituting an antiarrhythmic agent, reversible causes (hyperthyroidism, hypertension, heart failure, cardiac surgery, pulmonary embolism) need to be addressed.

Antiarrhythmic agents are divided into classes according to mechanism of action. Class I agents are sodium channel blockers and prolong the QT interval, leading to the potential for proarrhythmia and torsades de pointes. Class Ia agents, which include quinidine, procainamide, and disopyramide, block potassium channels as well. Quinidine can cause sinus and AV nodal blockade, in addition to its proarrhythmic effects. When initiating this agent the patient should have continuous ECG monitoring. Non-cardiac effects include abdominal cramping, nausea, and diarrhea, and cinchonism, a constellation of symptoms (tinnitus, hearing loss, blurred vision, delirium, confusion, and psychosis) associated with high plasma levels of the drug. Procainamide side effects include lupus-like syndrome, nausea, vomiting dizziness, psychosis, headache, depression, vasculitis, myalgias, fever, and pancytopenia or agranulocytosis, which may be life-threatening. Procainamide can also lengthen the PR interval in patients with AV conduction disease. The drug has an active metabolite (N-acetylprocainamide), and should be adjusted in renal or hepatic impairment. Disopyramide has negative inotropic effects and should be avoided in patients with heart failure, and is anticholinergic symptoms and should not be used in patients with glaucoma, myasthenia gravis, or urinary retention. Disopyramide needs to be adjusted for renal and hepatic impairment.

Class Ic antiarrhythmic agents (flecainide, propafenone, moricizine) block sodium channels but have less profound effects on repolarization. All class Ic agents have a negative inotropic effect and therefore are contraindicated in patients with heart failure. Extracardiac effects of flecainide include dizziness, headache, blurred vision, and ataxia. Propafenone has β-blocking effects in addition to class Ic antiarrhythmic properties, and should be avoided in patients with reactive airway diseases and sinus node dysfunction. Other common side effects include nausea, metallic taste, increased liver enzymes, dizziness, and constipation.

Class III antiarrhythmic agents (amiodarone, sotalol, dofetilide, ibutilide) are potassium channel blockers and prolong repolarization, action potential durations and refractory periods. All class III agents increase the QT interval and may precipitate torsades de pointes. Amiodarone blocks potassium, sodium, and calcium channels, and α- and β-receptors. Amiodarone is highly lipid soluble and accumulates in high concentrations in adipose tissue and highly perfused organs, such as the lung, liver, and skin. Because of the extensive accumulation the elimination half-life is long after discontinuation of the drug. The adverse effects of amiodarone therapy include pulmonary fibrosis, thyroid dysfunction, AV node blockade, hepatotoxicity, corneal microdeposits, optic nerve injury, gray-blue skin discoloration, tremor, ataxia, and peripheral neuropathy. Amiodarone interacts with other drugs, notably warfarin and digoxin, mandating dose adjustments if taken together. Liver function tests, thyroid function tests, and pulmonary function should be monitored periodically in patients on amiodarone (Goldschlager et al., 2000). Sotalol is a racemic mixture of D- and L-isomers that has class III and β-blocker actions. Side effects are largely due to the β-blockade, mandating caution in patients with reactive airway disease, sinus bradycardia, AV block. and uncontrolled heart failure. Sotalol has proarrhythmic affects and should not be administered to patients with prolonged QT intervals; initiation of sotalol is performed in a hospital setting with continuous cardiac monitoring. Sotalol is excreted by the kidneys and the dose should be adjusted in renal impairment. Dofetilide blocks the rapid component of the delayed rectifier potassium current, and prolongs the repolarization and refractory period in the atrium and ventricles without affecting the conduction system. Dofetilide prolongs the QT interval, and poses a risk of developing torsades de pointes, which is greatest within the first 3 days of drug initiation, so the drug is started in the hospital with continuous cardiac monitoring. Dofetilide is renally eliminated and interacts with a number of drugs, including verapamil, cimetidine, diuretics, ketoconazole, macrolide antibiotics, trimethoprim, triamterene, metformin, amiloride, and megestrol. Ibutilide is an intravenous class III antiarrhythmic drug that is used to terminate acute atrial fibrillation acutely. One milligram of ibutilide should be infused over 10 minutes. Termination of the arrhythmia should occur with 60 minutes of initiating the dose, and if the arrhythmia does not terminate the dose may be repeated. Like all class III agents, ibutilide can lengthen the QT interval and precipitate torsades de pointes, and so continuous ECG monitoring for 6 hours after drug administration is mandatory, even if sinus rhythm has been restored.

The choice of an antiarrhythmic agent depends on the clinical setting. Propafenone or flecainide are recommended as first-line drugs for pharmacological cardioversion in patients without structural heart disease, although amiodarone, sotalol, and dofetilide are alternative agents (Fuster et al., 2001). Sotalol and amiodarone can be used for adrenergically mediated atrial fibrillation, and disopyramide is suggested for vagally induced atrial fibrillation. In patients with structural heart disease, amiodarone and sotalol are recommended as the first line drugs. Class Ic antiarrhythmic agents (flecainide, encainide, moricizine) should be avoided in patients with coronary heart disease owing to the increased mortality shown in the Cardiac Arrhythmia Suppression Trial (CAST II Investigators, 1992; Echt et al., 1991) Amiodarone is recommended for patients with heart failure and atrial fibrillation; dofetilide is an alternative (Fuster et al., 2001).

The other important issue in the management of patients with atrial fibrillation is prevention of complications, most notably stroke. Atrial fibrillation is a risk factor for stroke, but varies among patients. The annual risk in the Framingham study was 4.2% but may be higher for patients with more than one risk factor (Wolf et al., 1978). Two studies, Atrial Fibrillation Investigation (AFI) (Atrial Fibrillation Investigators, 1994) and Stroke Prevention in Atrial Fibrillation (SPAF)

(Hart et al., 1999) identified individual risk factors that increased the risk of stroke in patients with atrial fibrillation. Risk factors for stroke in the AFI study included previous stroke, hypertension, diabetes, and advanced age. SPAF correlated stroke risk with previous stroke, females over the age 75, systolic hypertension, and low ejection fraction (EF). To simplify the system, Gage et al. (2001) combined the risk factors from both studies and devised a point system called CHADS2. Two points were given to a history of previous stroke, and all other risk factors were given 1 point. A score of 0–1 was identified as low risk for stroke and warfarin was not recommended. A score of 2–3 was moderate risk, 4–6 was high risk. Warfarin was recommended for both the moderate and high-risk groups.

The ACC/AHA/ESC developed their own risk-based approach to antithrombotic therapy in patients with atrial fibrillation (Table 1). These guidelines recommend warfarin for patients with atrial fibrillation and valvular disease, previous stroke, or at least one risk factor (heart failure, female over the age of 75, low EF, diabetes, hypertension). Aspirin is recommended for patients less than 60 years old with no risk factors with or without heart disease and patients older than 60 years with no heart disease and no risk factors. The target international normalized ratio range for nonvalvular atrial fibrillation is 2–3, and 2.5–3.5 for valvular disease (Fuster et al., 2001).

Whether anticoagulation can be stopped in patients who have converted to sinus rhythm is a difficult and unresolved question. The results of the rate-control versus rhythm-control strategies described earlier suggest that patients who have been converted to sinus rhythm may have paroxysmal episodes of atrial fibrillation that go undetected. On the other hand, anticoagulation poses a risk of hemorrhage. In general, chronic anticoagulation with warfarin is desirable unless the patient is a low risk for stroke or the drug is contraindicated (Snow et al., 2003).

Nonpharmacological therapies (surgical ablation, percutaneous catheter ablation) are indicated for patients who are symptomatic and refractory to medical therapy. Foci in the pulmonary veins, superior vena cava, right and left atrium or coronary sinus can be ablated percutaneously using a radiofrequency catheter. The risk of recurrence after focal ablation is currently about is 30–50%, and many patients still require antiarrhythmic therapy after ablation (Fuster et al., 2001). Complications of catheter ablation include

Table 1
Risk-Based Approach to Antithrombotic Therapy in Patients With Atrial Fibrillation

Patient features	Antithrombotic therapy
Age <60, no heart disease	Aspirin 325 mg per day or no therapy
Age <60, heart disease but no risk factors [a]	Aspirin 325 mg per day
Age >60, no risk factors [a]	Aspirin 325 mg per day
Age >60 with diabetes or CAD	Warfarin (INR 2–3)
	Addition of aspirin, 81–162 mg per day is optional
Age >75, especially women	Warfarin (INR approximately 2)
Heart failure (EF <35%)	Warfarin (INR 2–3)
Thyrotoxicosis	
Hypertension	
Rheumatic heart disease	Warfarin (INR 2.5–3.5)
Prosthetic heart valves	
Prior thromboembolism	
Persistent atrial thrombus on TEE	

[a] Risk factors for thromboembolism include heart failure, ejection fraction less than 35%, and a history of hypertension.

INR, international normalized ratio; CAD, coronary artery disease; EF, ejection fraction; TEE, transesophageal echocardiography.

Adapted from Fuster et al. (2001).

pulmonary vein stenosis, pericardial effusion and tamponade, phrenic nerve paralysis, and systemic embolism. Catheter ablation of the AV node with insertion of a permanent pacemaker is another option. A meta-analysis concluded that AV nodal ablation and pacemaker implantation improved symptoms, quality of life, exercise duration, and LV function (Wood et al., 2000). Surgical ablation, the Maze procedure, is an invasive approach that requires a thoracotomy and general anesthesia. This option is usually employed in patients requiring open heart surgery for other indications.

SUPRAVENTRICULAR TACHYCARDIA

Sinus Tachycardia

Sinus tachycardia is a rhythm that arises from the sinoatrial (SA) node with a heart rate of more than 100 bpm. It is usually a physiological response to an underlying cause, which can include pain, anxiety, fever, exercise, hyperthyroidism, volume depletion, hypotension, pulmonary embolism, MI, anemia, or infection. Certain illicit drugs, such as cocaine, amphetamines, and ecstasy can precipitate this arrhythmia. Other stimulants (caffeine, alcohol, nicotine) and prescribed medications (atropine, catecholamines, aminophylline, doxorubicin, daunorubicin) can induce sinus tachycardia.

Occasional patients may have inappropriate sinus tachycardia, an uncommon arrhythmia that occurs most commonly in young women, a disproportionate number from the health care profession. The mechanism is unclear; studies have suggested that there is abnormal sinus node automaticity or excess sympathetic and reduced parasympathetic tone (Bauernfeind et al., 1979; Blomstrom-Lundqvist et al., 2003). Diagnostic criteria include exclusion of secondary causes.

Patients may be asymptomatic or may complain of palpitations, lightheadedness, or dizziness. The P-waves have be the same sinus morphology (upright in leads I, II, and III). With increasing heart rate, the PR interval decreases. The QRS complex is narrow. Vagal maneuvers (carotid massage or Valsalva maneuver) may help in differentiating sinus tachycardia from other paroxysmal supraventricular tachycardias.

The first priority in the treatment of sinus tachycardia is to identify the underlying cause. Once the cause is identified, treatment can be tailored to that cause. Pharmacological therapy can be used in certain situations. β-Blockers may be used to treat sinus tachycardia resulting from anxiety, hyperthyroidism, and MI. For in appropriate sinus tachycardia, β-blockers are first-line therapy, with CCBs as an alternative (Blomstrom-Lundqvist et al., 2003) if β-blockers are contraindicated. If patients are refractory to medical therapy, sinus node modification by catheter ablation is an option.

Focal (Ectopic) Atrial Tachycardia

Repetitive focal atrial tachycardia is thought to be caused by enhanced automaticity arising from a single atrial focus. This arrhythmia is seen in patients with organic heart disease, lung disease, MI, infection, electrolyte disturbances (hypokalemia), and hypoxemia. Medications that can enhance automaticity include digoxin and theophylline. Drugs of abuse such as cocaine and alcohol can also induce this arrhythmia.

On the ECG, the P-wave morphology will be consistent but different from the sinus P-waves. The QRS complex is usually narrow. There is often a progressive acceleration in the atrial rate (warm up) at the beginning followed by a gradual decrease at the end of the arrhythmia (cool down).

For acute treatment in hemodynamically stable patients, either adenosine, β-blockers or conversion with intravenous antiarrhythmics from classes Ia, Ic, or III is recommended (Blomstrom-Lundqvist et al., 2003). Hemodynamically unstable patients should be cardioverted. If rate regulation only is needed in the acute setting, intravenous β-blockers, verapamil, or diltiazem is indicated. Digoxin can also be used as long as the arrhythmia is not the result of digoxin toxicity. For prophylactic therapy to prevent recurrence, β-blockers and CCBs are the treatment of choice. Disopyramide, flecainide, propafenone, sotalol, and amiodarone are alternatives for prophylactic treatment (Blomstrom-Lundqvist et al., 2003). Class Ic antiarrhythmics should not be given to patients with CAD. For symptomatic patients refractory to medical therapy, catheter ablation is recommended.

Multifocal Atrial Tachycardia

Multifocal atrial tachycardia (MAT) usually occurs in the acutely ill, elderly patient, or in those with pulmonary disease (McCord &

Borzak, 1998). MAT is also associated with diabetes, hypokalemia, hypomagnesemia, chronic kidney disease, hypoxia, acidosis, hypercapnia, and certain medications. MAT is diagnosed by the presence of three or more different P-wave morphologies on one ECG with an irregularly irregular rhythm. The most useful therapy for MAT is to treat the underlying causes, including hypoxemia and hypercapnia, myocardial ischemia, congestive heart failure, or electrolyte disturbances. β-Blockers and CCBs can slow an excessive ventricular rate (Levine et al., 1985). These agents should be used cautiously in patients with known congestive heart failure or reduced LV function.

AV Nodal Reentry Tachycardia

Atrioventricular nodal reentry tachycardia (AVNRT) is the most common paroxysmal supraventricular tachycardia, accounting for about 60% of all supraventricular arrhythmias (Kastor, 1994). It tends to be more common in women than men. Symptoms emerge most commonly in young adults, although they can occur at any age. Most patients with AVNRT do not have structural heart disease.

Dual AV nodal pathways with different conduction velocities and refractory periods are usually present, setting up the substrate for reentry (Mazgalev & Tchou, 2000). The slow pathway has a short refractory time, and the fast pathway has a longer refractory time. A normal sinus beat travels down both fast and slow pathways. In the most common variant, slow–fast AVNRT, a critically timed premature beat finds that the fast pathway is still refractory, and conducts down the slow pathway. If the fast pathway has recovered, the impulse can then be conducted retrograde up the fast pathway to the atrium, creating a re-entrant circuit. The uncommon fast-slow AVNRT has antegrade conduction down the fast pathway and retrograde conduction up the slow pathway.

The symptoms of AVNRT are related to the rapid heart rate and include palpitations, lightheadedness, dizziness, and sometimes syncope. Some patients may experience chest pain or dyspnea. The heart rate ranges from 120 to 220 bpm. The P-wave can occur immediately before or after the QRS complex, or may not be seen on the ECG because of near-simultaneous retrograde atrial and antegrade ventricular activation. If P-wave occurs immediately after the QRS, there may be a pseudo-R-wave in V1 or pseudo-S-wave leads II, III, and aVF reflecting retrograde conduction. In the less common fast–slow AVNRT, the P-wave may occur just before the next QRS.

Carotid sinus massage or other vagal maneuvers may convert AVNRT to normal sinus rhythm. Adenosine 6 to 12 mg intravenously is the preferred initial drug treatment because its extremely short half-life minimizes side effects. The 12 mg dose may be repeated if necessary. Urgent cardioversion may be necessary with circulatory insufficiency. The AV node action potential is calcium channel-dependent, which make verapamil or diltiazem very effective in terminating this arrhythmia. β-Blockers are also effective.

For chronic therapy in patients with frequent symptomatic episodes, β-blockers are preferred because they suppress the initiating premature atrial contractions. CCBs and digoxin can also be used. In patients who do not respond to AV nodal blocking agents and who do not have structural heart disease, flecainide or propafenone are the recommended antiarrhythmic drugs of choice (Blomstrom-Lundqvist et al., 2003).

Radiofrequency catheter ablation of the slow pathway is a curative treatment modality in patients with AVNRT. In the North American Society for Pacing and Electrophysiology prospective registry, the success rate was 96.1%, with AV block as a complication in only 1% (Scheinman & Huang, 2000). Based on these results, and with appropriate selection by physicians, many patients with recurrent AVNRT are choosing catheter ablation therapy over antiarrhythmic therapy.

Atrioventricular Reciprocating Tachycardia

Atrioventricular reciprocating tachycardia (AVRT) is characterized by an extra-nodal accessory bypass tract connecting the atrium to the ventricles. Approximately 30% of patients with supraventricular tachycardia will be found to have an accessory pathway (Kastor, 1994).

Conduction through these accessory pathways can be from the atrium to the ventricles (antegrade conduction) or from the ventricles to the atrium (retrograde conduction). When conduction goes down the AV node and back up the bypass tract, the QRS complex is narrow and conduction is termed *orthodromic* (Kastor, 1994). When conduction goes down the bypass tract and back up the AV node, the QRS complex is wide and conduction is termed *antidromic* (Kastor, 1994).

Accessory pathways that are capable of antegrade conduction pre-excite the ventricles. The characteristic ECG finding of this pre-excitation is the delta wave. Patients with a delta wave and an AVRT are said to have Wolff-Parkinson-White (WPW) syndrome. There are no characteristic ECG findings when the accessory pathway conducts in the retrograde direction. These pathways are termed *concealed accessory pathways*.

In AVRT, a critically timed premature atrial or ventricular beat initiates a reentrant tachycardia. Orthodromic AVRT uses the AV node and His-Purkinje system to conduct the impulse to the ventricles; the QRS complex is narrow, and the heart rate ranges from 150 to 250 bpm. In antidromic AVRT, the impulses are conducted to the ventricle through the accessory pathway, generating a wide QRS complex. Antidromic AVRT is faster because of the relatively short refractory period of the accessory pathway.

Wolff-Parkinson-White Syndrome

WPW syndrome is a pre-excitation syndrome characterized by an accessory pathway (bundle of Kent) that bypasses the AV node and activates the ventricles prematurely. Most patients with WPW have otherwise normal hearts, but some have congenital anomalies, such as Ebstein's anomaly, septal defects, transposition of the great vessels, and a familial form of hypertrophic cardiomyopathy. The prevalence of WPW syndrome is approximately 0.1–0.3% of the general population. WPW is twice as common in men as in women.

The ECG findings include a shortened PR interval, delta wave and a widened QRS complex. The PR interval is short owing to the rapid AV conduction through the accessory pathway, bypassing the delay in the AV node. The delta wave is produced by the slow early activation of the ventricles by the accessory pathway. The widened QRS complex results from fusion of early ventricular activation by the accessory pathway and activation from the impulses conducted through the AV node and infranodal system.

Most patients with WPW syndrome present with symptoms of tachyarrhythmias. Tachyarrhythmias associated with WPW syndrome include AVRT, atrial fibrillation, atrial flutter, and ventricular fibrillation. Approximately 10–30% of patients with WPW will develop atrial fibrillation (Campbell et al., 1977). In those patients, AVRT usual precedes atrial fibrillation. The impulses generated during atrial fibrillation can conduct antegrade down the accessory pathway, and can be transmitted at very high rates (>250 bpm) due to the short refractory time of the accessory pathway.

The ECG in atrial fibrillation with WPW is characteristic. The diagnosis is made by the irregularly irregular rhythm, which indicates atrial fibrillation, and the varying width of the QRS complexes, which is caused by varying degrees of fusion resulting from antegrade conduction down both the normal conducting system and the bypass tract. Some of the R-R intervals can be extremely short, less than 250 ms. Rapid atrial fibrillation in WPW is very dangerous because it can deteriorate to ventricular fibrillation and sudden cardiac death.

THERAPY

Pharmacological treatment of AVRT must be tailored to the electrophysiological properties of the arrhythmia. Therapy of orthodromic accessory pathway reentrant tachycardias entails AV nodal blockade with vagal maneuvers, IV adenosine, and CCBs (Blomstrom-Lundqvist et al., 2003). Second-line drugs include intravenous procainamide and β-blockers. Chronic therapy for orthodromic AVRT usually involves administration of class Ic antiarrhythmic drugs (flecainide, encainide).

For antidromic accessory pathway reentrant tachycardias, intravenous procainamide is the drug of choice because it slows conduction down the accessory pathway. Atrial flutter or fibrillation with antidromic conduction is a dangerous situation due to the potential for extremely rapid conduction down the accessory pathway with resultant rapid ventricular rates. In this situation, the ventricular rate is modulated by competition between AV nodal conduction and conduction down the bypass tract. Drugs that block the AV node such as digoxin, verapamil, or diltiazem can thus increase ventricular rate and lead to the potential for ventricular fibrillation. In both orthodromic and antidromic AVRT, cardioversion is indicated for hemodynamic collapse.

For chronic therapy of antidromic AVRT, class Ic antiarrhythmic drugs are recommended (Blomstrom-Lundqvist et al., 2003). Amiodarone and class Ia agents can be used as second-line therapy.

Catheter ablation is potentially curative, and has a low complication rate (Jackman et al., 1991; Wang & Yao, 2003). Catheter ablation was given a class I recommendation by the ACC/AHA/ESC for patients with WPW syndrome and symptomatic arrhythmias, atrial fibrillation or poorly tolerated AVRT (Blomstrom-Lundqvist et al., 2003). The same group gave catheter ablation a class IIa recommendation for asymptomatic patients in high-risk occupations. Many patients with recurrent arrhythmias choose catheter ablation over lifelong antiarrhythmic medication, although recurrences after ablation do occur (Wang & Yao, 2003).

Junctional Tachycardia

Junctional tachycardias are rare and usually benign. They result from increased automaticity arising from a high junctional focus or triggered activity (Lee et al., 1999). Nonparoxysmal junctional tachycardia is usually caused by digoxin toxicity, hypokalemia, theophylline, inferior wall MIs, myocarditis, catecholamine excess, or postcardiac surgery.

The ECG shows a narrow complex tachycardia with absent P-waves and a heart rate ranging from 70 to 110 bom. Onset is usually gradual with a typical "warm-up" and "cool-down" pattern. If digoxin toxicity is the etiology, the ECG may show a second-degree Mobitz type I block.

Management for junctional tachycardia is to eliminate and correct the underlying cause. Occasionally, loss of AV synchrony leads to decreased cardiac output. Overdrive atrial pacing at an appropriate rate can improve AV synchrony and cardiac output. Persistent junctional tachycardia can be treated with β-blockers or CCBs (Lee et al., 1999).

VENTRICULAR TACHYCARDIA

Ventricular tachyarrhythmias can be classified as benign or malignant. The chief distinction, in addition to duration and hemodynamic consequences, is the presence of significant structural heart disease. This distinction is especially important when evaluating premature ventricular contractions (PVCs) and nonsustained ventricular tachycardia (NSVT). In patients without structural heart disease, the risk of sudden death or hemodynamic compromise is minimal, and therapy is rarely necessary in the absence of symptoms. In patients with CAD, a history of MI, or cardiomyopathy, PVCs may indicate the potential for malignant ventricular tachyarrhythmias and merit prompt and thorough assessment. Prompt evaluation for and reversal of precipitating factors such as ischemia and electrolyte abnormalities are indicated.

Ventricular tachycardia can be monomorphic or polymorphic, sustained or nonsustained. Sustained ventricular tachycardia is defined as persisting for longer than 30 seconds; nonsustained has at least three or more ventricular beats but lasts less than 30 seconds.

The signs and symptoms of ventricular dysrhythmia range from palpitations, diaphoresis, dizziness, lightheadedness, shortness of breath, chest pain, pre-syncope, syncope, and sudden cardiac death. Some patients may be completely asymptomatic. A complete history and physical exam should be performed on all patients with ventricular dysrhythmias. The patient should be questioned about a family history of sudden cardiac death and evaluated for risk factors of CAD.

Ventricular tachycardia is a wide complex rhythm that must be distinguished from supraventricular tachycardia with aberrant conduction. Clues that suggest a ventricular origin include AV dissociation, fusion beats (which result from simultaneous activation of two foci, one ventricular and one supraventricular), and capture beats (beats that capture the ventricle and are conducted with a narrow complex, ruling out fixed bundle branch block), as well as severe left axis deviation ($-60°$ to $120°$). A more systematic approach to distinguish ventricular tachycardia from a wide-complex supraventricular tachycardia was outlined by Brugada et al. (1991) The diagnosis is ventricular tachycardia if there is absence of the RS complex in all precordial leads, R to S interval is greater than 100 ms in one precordial lead, AV dissociation, or characteristic morphology in leads V_1, V_2, and V_6. If not, the arrhythmia is most likely supraventricular tachycardia with aberrant conduction.

Sustained monomorphic ventricular tachycardia is a reentrant rhythm most commonly occurring more than 48 hours after an MI, or in the setting of cardiomyopathy. Initial management of sustained monomorphic ventricular tachycardia with a history of structural heart disease depends on its rate, duration, and hemodynamic status. Unstable ventricular tachycardia is an indication for prompt defibrillation. Hemodynamically stable patients with a risk of imminent circulatory collapse may be treated with an antiarrhythmic such as intravenous amiodarone. Current Advanced Cardiac Life Support guidelines consider lidocaine and intravenous procainamide alternative choices. If the arrhythmia recurs, intravenous antiarrhythmic drug therapy, with either amiodarone, lidocaine, or procainamide, should be initiated.

Enthusiasm for the use of chronic antiarrhythmic agents to prevent ventricular arrhythmias was considerably dampened after the CAST, which showed an increase in mortality in patients receiving flecainide or encainide in patients with CAD (Echt et al., 1991). There has been concern that other antiarrhythmic agents could have the same proarrhythmic effects. Available data suggests that amiodarone and sotalol are the most effective antiarrhythmic drugs for preventing sustained ventricular tachycardia.

Clinical trials comparing insertion of automated implantable cardioverter defibrillators (AICD) to antiarrhythmic drug therapy have generally shown a benefit for AICD placement. In high-risk patients (NSVT, prior Q-wave MI, EF of 35% or less, inducible sustained ventricular tachycardia not suppressed by procainamide at electrophysiological study), the Multicenter Automatic Defibrillator Implantation Trial (MADIT) study showed significantly improved survival with AICD compared to conventional medical therapy (Moss et al., 1996). Similarly, the Antiarrhythmics Versus Implantable Defibrillator (AVID) study showed that patients resuscitated from ventricular fibrillation or with hemodynamically significant ventricular tachycardia with EF of 40% or less had improved survival with AICD compared to antiarrhythmic therapy (amiodarone in more than 80%) (AVID Investigators, 1997).

AICD placement appears to be effective as primary prevention as well. The MADIT-II trial demonstrated that prophylactic placement of an implantable cardioverter defibrillator (ICD) in patients with LVEF of 30% or less after MI improved survival (Moss et al., 2002). The timing of ICD implantation however, is uncertain. In the recent Defibrillator in Acute Myocardial Infarction, placement of an ICD immediately after an MI did not reduce all-cause mortality (Hohnloser et al., 2004), and analysis of MADIT-II demonstrated that patients with a remote MI (at least 18 months previous) benefited greatly from the ICD, whereas those with a more recent MI (<18 months) did not (Greenberg et al., 2004). Data from the Sudden

Cardiac Death-Heart Failure trial also showed a survival benefit in patients with either an ischemic or a non-ischemic cardiomyopathy and EF less than 35% after implantation of an AICD compared to amiodarone (Bardy et al., 2005). Because of the outcomes of these trials, implantable defibrillators are recommended for survivors of sudden cardiac death and patients with a previous MI and LVEF of less than 35%.

The challenge in selecting patients for AICD implantation is that identification of the highest risk subgroups leads to very cost-effective use of devices but identifies only a small proportion of the 300,000 sudden cardiac deaths that occur annually in the United States (Myerburg et al., 1998). Improvement in risk-stratification techniques and strategies to consider costs and benefits in the general population is driving the evolution of AICD use in the community.

Torsade de Pointes

Torsade de pointes is a syndrome consisting of polymorphic ventricular tachycardia with QT prolongation. Polymorphic ventricular tachycardia without QT prolongation most commonly occurs in the setting of acute myocardial ischemia. Although polymorphic ventricular tachycardia is often faster than sustained monomorphic ventricular tachycardia and thus can lead to hemodynamic instability, many episodes of polymorphic ventricular tachycardia terminate spontaneously. Initial management for polymorphic ventricular tachycardia without QT prolongation is similar to that for monomorphic ventricular tachycardia, with defibrillation and antiarrhythmic drugs (Grogin & Scheinman, 1993).

Torsade de pointes can occur in the absence of structural heart disease. Acquired QT prolongation is most often caused by drugs, including type I and type III antiarrhythmic agents, tricyclic antidepressants, phenothiazines, nonsedating antihistamines, erythromycin, pentamidine, and azole antifungal agents. QT prolongation may also be caused by electrolyte abnormalities, especially hypomagnesemia, and exacerbated by other conditions such as hypothyroidism, cerebrovascular accident, and liquid protein diets (Napolitano et al., 1994).

Torsade de pointes is triggered by early afterdepolarizations, oscillations in the membrane potential that occur during prolonged repolarization, usually in the setting of an accumulation of intracellular positive ions. This abnormality can occur from malfunctioning ion channels, electrolyte disruptions, or by medications, and may be exacerbated by increased sympathetic activity. The early after depolarizations depolarize nearby cell membranes, which can results in action potentials, initiating polymorphic ventricular tachycardia.

The ECG of torsade de pointes will show a beat-to-beat change in the QRS axis, irregular RR intervals, and a heart rate ranging from 160 to 250 bpm. A pause may be seen before the onset of torsade. Ventricular bigeminy in a patient with a long QT interval may be a sign of impending torsade. On the resting ECG, The QT interval varies inversely with the heart rate and therefore must be corrected, usually using Bazett's formula, in which the corrected QT interval (QTc) is the QT interval divided by the square root of the RR interval in milliseconds. A QTc of more than 0.44 seconds in men and more than 0.45 seconds in women is considered prolonged.

Empiric magnesium (2 g intravenously over 1 to 2 minutes) should be given to all patients with suspected torsade de pointes because the risk is low and the potential benefits high. Because the length of the QT interval is affected by the RR interval, use of isoproterenol or temporary pacing in patients with acquired QT prolongation and torsade de pointes to increase the heart rate can be effective (Roden, 1993). Nonsynchronized electrical defibrillation may be required in hemodynamically unstable patients.

Long QT Syndrome

Congenital long QT (LQT) syndrome is a disorder of ventricular repolarization characterized by a prolonged QT interval. This prolongation of the QT interval predisposes the patient to torsade de pointes, ventricular fibrillation and sudden cardiac death. Forms of congenital LQT syndrome include Jervell and Lange-Nielsen syndrome, which is associated with sensorineural deafness, and Romano-Ward syndrome. Genes responsible for LQT syndrome have been identified and the syndrome classified into subtypes according to mutation. Of the two most common mutations, LQT type I is associated with mutations in KVLQT1, an outward-rectifying cardiac potassium channel protein, LQT type 2 with mutations in the human ether-related-a-go-go (*HERG*) gene, another component of the outward-rectifying potassium channel, and LQT type 3 with mutations in the cardiac sodium channel gene *SCN5A*. This is important because these three subtypes have different arrhythmic triggers and respond differently to medications. LQT syndrome is perhaps the best example of the use of genotyping to guide prognosis and therapy in current cardiological practice.

The signs and symptoms of congenital LQT syndrome occur during childhood or adolescence. Syncope or cardiac arrest during physical exertion or emotional stress may be the first presenting symptom. Arrhythmic events in patients with LQT1 are most often related to exercise, and also with swimming. Events triggered by auditory stimuli, such as alarm clocks and telephones, are most typically seen in patients with LQT2. Patients with LQT3 are at highest risk of events when at rest or asleep. The clinical course of LQT syndrome is also influenced by genotype; patients with LQT1 tend to have the earliest events and a worse prognosis, and those with LQT3 have a later onset and a lower overall event rate. There is also a difference in clinical course with different mutations within one subtype.

The mainstay of pharmacological therapy for congenital LQT syndrome is β-blockade, titrated to blunt the maximum heart rate achieved by exertion. Competitive sports should be avoided. The efficacy of β-blockers varies with genotype; they are most effective in patients with LQT1, and least effective in patients with LQT3. Left cardiac sympathetic denervation is occasionally performed to prevent cardiac events. Cardiac pacing has been employed in patients who remain symptomatic despite medical therapy, and may be especially useful in patients with LQT3. AICD implantation is recommended in patients who have recurrent syncope, sustained ventricular arrhythmias, or sudden cardiac death despite drug therapy (Antzelevitch et al., 2005; Gregoratos et al., 1998).

Arrhythmogenic Right Ventricular Dysplasia

Arrhythmogenic right ventricular dysplasia (ARVD) is a myocardial disorder in which there is replacement of the right ventricle myocardium with fatty or fibrofatty tissue, with the potential for a reentrant ventricular tachycardia and sudden death. ARVD occurs in families, with both an autosomal dominant and autosomal recessive form. A familial form of ARVD accompanied by hyperkeratosis and woolly hair with autosomal recessive inheritance was identified on a Greek island and termed Naxos disease.

The clinical manifestations include palpitations, dizziness, syncope, right-sided heart failure, sustained or nonsustained monomorphic ventricular tachycardia and sudden cardiac death. The ECG is characteristic, includes a prolonged QRS complex with a right bundle branch pattern, ε wave (electric potentials after the end of the QRS complex) and T-wave inversions in leads V_1 to V_3. Diagnostic testing includes echocardiography, signal-averaged ECG, and magnetic resonance imaging, which is the best method to demonstrate fatty infiltration of the right ventricular (RV) myocardium. Signal-averaged ECG may be used to screen family members.

Both ventricular tachycardia and sudden death can be exercise-induced, possibly due to RV stress and catecholamine stimulation, and so patients with ARVD should not participate in competitive sports. Therapy should be aimed at suppression of arrhythmias. Sotalol is the most effective antiarrhythmic medication for suppressing ventricular arrhythmias in ARVD. Amiodarone is the second choice. Implantable defibrillators are indicated (class I) for symptomatic patients and survivors of sudden cardiac death, and may be considered (class IIa) for secondary prevention and a class IIa for primary prevention of ventricular tachycardia in ARVD (Priori et al., 2001). Ablation of arrhythmic foci has been undertaken, but ARVD tends to progress, and so this therapy is usually reserved for patients with non-life-threatening but symptomatic tachyarrhythmias who are intolerant of antiarrhythmic drugs.

Brugada Syndrome

Brugada syndrome is a rare genetic disease that is characterized by ST elevation unrelated to electrolyte disorders or coronary ischemia. Brugada syndrome can cause sudden cardiac death from ventricular fibrillation in individuals with structurally normal hearts. The ECG findings are distinctive, and include a pseudo-right bundle branch block pattern with ST elevation in leads V_1 through V_3. Cases of Brugada syndrome have now been linked with mutations in the cardiac sodium channel gene *SCN5A* (Chen et al., 1998). There is some suggestion that Brugada syndrome may be an early manifestation of arrhythmogenic RV dysplasia, but this is uncertain.

The diagnosis of Brugada syndrome relies on the ECG findings and the clinical presentation. The diagnosis of Brugada syndrome should be considered if the patient has coved type ST segment elevation in more than one precordial lead and one of the following: documented ventricular fibrillation, self-terminating polymorphic ventricular tachycardia, a family history of sudden cardiac death at age less than 45 years old, coved ST segment elevation in family members, electrophysiological inducibility, syncope, and nocturnal agonal respiration (Wilde et al., 2002). A patient with ECG findings without clinical manifestations is defined as having Brugada pattern (Wilde et al., 2002).

There are no well-established pharmacological therapies. β-Blockers and amiodarone have not been shown to be beneficial. There is some suggestion that quinidine may be useful (Belhassen et al., 2004).

Implantation of an AICD is the only currently proven therapy to prevent sudden death, and is recommended in patients with syncope, symptomatic ventricular tachycardia, or a prior history of aborted sudden cardiac death (Gregoratos et al., 1998; Priori et al., 2001). What to do with asymptomatic patients is less certain. Stratification by electrophysiological testing, with AICD implantation in patients with inducible ventricular tachycardia, has been advocated (Antzelevitch et al., 2005).

Bradycardias

Sinus Node Dysfunction

Bradycardias associated with sinus node dysfunction include sinus bradycardia, sinus pause, SA block, and sinus arrest. These disturbances often result from increased vagal tone (Atlee, 1997). If bradycardia is transient and not associated with hemodynamic compromise, no therapy is necessary. If bradycardia is sustained or compromises end-organ perfusion, therapy with antimuscarinic agents, such as atropine, or β-agonists such as ephedrine may be initiated. Transcutaneous or transvenous pacing may be necessary in some cases.

Patients with a combination of bradycardia with paroxysmal atrial tachycardias owing to pre-existing conduction system disease can be challenging to manage pharmacologically. In these cases, insertion of a temporary pacemaker may allow the administration of rate-lowering agents.

Heart Block

The most common cause of acquired chronic AV heart block is fibrosis of the conducting system. Although pre-existing conduction system disease is a risk factor for the development of complete heart block, no single laboratory or clinical variable identifies patients at risk for progression to high-degree AV block (Gregoratos et al., 1998). In first-degree AV block there is prolongation of conduction time of the atrial impulses to the ventricles, with a PR interval greater than 200 ms. In second-degree AV block, conducted atrial beats are interspersed with nonconducted beats. Second-degree AV block is divided into Mobitz type I (Wenckebach) and Mobitz type II block. In Mobitz I block, the PR interval lengthens progressively until the P-wave fails to conduct. In most cases, the block occurs at the AV node. Mobitz I block can occur in healthy individuals, the elderly, and in patients with underlying heart disease. In Mobitz type II AV block the PR interval remains constant until a P-wave fails to conduct. Mobitz II block occurs below the AV node, and thus is more dangerous since it is much more likely to progress to complete heart block. In third-degree AV block, none of the atrial impulses are conducted to the ventricles. The escape rhythm, whether junctional or ventricular, is generally regular.

Patients with AV block may be asymptomatic, but may experience dizziness or syncope as a consequence of decreased cardiac output. AV block is most commonly caused by AV nodal conduction disease, but AV nodal-blocking agents need to be ruled out as causative agents. Any medications that affect conduction through the AV node should be decreased or discontinued if possible.

Recommendations for pacemaker implantation differ a bit among societies, but in general are predicated on symptoms and the potential for progression to higher degrees of heart block. A pacemaker is generally not recommended in most cases of first-degree AV block, although it may be considered in patients with marked PR prolongation (>300 ms) and LV dysfunction with heart failure symptoms (Gregoratos et al., 1998). A second- or third-degree block and either symptomatic bradycardia or congestive heart failure is a class I indication (general agreement that a treatment is beneficial) for insertion of a pacemaker (Gregoratos et al., 1998). The ACC/AHA/ NASPE have given permanent pacing for asymptomatic patients with Mobitz type II AV block a class IIa recommendation (conflict-

Table 2
Recommendations for Permanent Pacing
After the Acute Phase of Myocardial Infarction

Class I	• Persistent second-degree AV block in the His-Purkinje system with bilateral bundle branch block or complete heart block after acute myocardial infarction. • Transient advanced (second- or third-degree) infranodal AV block and associated bundle branch block. If the site of block is uncertain, an electrophysiological study may be necessary • Persistent and symptomatic second- or third-degree AV block.
Class IIb	• Persistent second- or third-degree AV block at the AV node level.
Class III	• Transient AV block in the absence of intraventricular conduction defects • Transient AV block in the presence of isolated left anterior fascicular block. • Acquired left anterior fascicular block in the absence of AV block. • Persistent first-degree AV block in the presence of bundle branch block that is old or age indeterminate.

Class I: evidence and/or general agreement that a treatment is beneficial; Class II: conflicting evidence, efficacy less well established; Class III: evidence and/or general agreement that a treatment is not useful and in some cases maybe harmful. (Adapted from Gregoratos et al., 2002.)

ing evidence, but weight of evidence favors usefulness) (Gregoratos et al., 1998). Permanent pacing was given a class I indication for all patients with third-degree or advanced heart block and either symptomatic bradycardia, pauses greater than 3 seconds, or escape rates less than 40 bpm. A class IIa recommendation for permanent pacing was given for patients with asymptomatic third-degree AV block (Gregoratos et al., 1998).

Pacemaker implantation is also indicated in patients who have bradycardia–tachycardia ("sick sinus") syndrome, and other arrhythmias or medical conditions that require drugs that result in symptomatic bradycardia (Gregoratos et al., 1998). Pacing may also be considered for patients with an inadequate chronotropic response to exercise.

Table 3
Recommendations for Temporary Transvenous
Pacing After an Acute Myocardial Infarction

Class I	• Asystole
	• Symptomatic bradycardia
	• Bilateral bundle branch block (alternating BBB or RBBB with alternating LAFB/LPFB, any age)
	• New or indeterminate-age bifascicular block (RBBB with LAFB or LPFB, or LBBB) with first-degree AV block
	• Mobitz type II second-degree AV block
Class IIa	• RBBB and LAFB or LPFB (new or indeterminate).
	• RBBB with first-degree AV block
	• LBBB, new or indeterminate.
	• Incessant VT, for atrial or ventricular overdrive pacing.
	• Recurrent sinus pauses (greater than 3 seconds) not responsive to atropine.
Class IIb	• Bifascicular block of indeterminate age.
	• New or age-indeterminate isolated RBBB.
Class III	• First-degree heart block.
	• Type I second-degree AV block with normal hemodynamics.
	• Accelerated idioventricular rhythm.
	• BBB or fascicular block known to exist before acute MI

RBBB, right bundle branch block; LBBB, left bundle branch block; LAFB, left anterior fascicular block; LPFV, left posterior fascicular block; AMI, acute myocardial infarction. Class I: evidence and/or general agreement that a treatment is beneficial; Class II: conflicting evidence; Class IIa:weight of evidence is in favor of efficacy; ClassIIb: weight of evidence is less well established; Class III: evidence and/or general agreement that a treatment is not useful and maybe harmful. (Adapted from Ryan et al., 1999.)

Conduction abnormalities are a common complication of acute MIs. These can be transient or permanent. Conduction abnormalities associated with an acute inferior MI usually result from AV nodal ischemia, are transient, and carry a low mortality rate. Conduction abnormalities in association with an acute anterior MI, however, represent extensive necrosis of the infranodal conduction system and the myocardium, and are associated with high in-hospital mortality (Hindman et al., 1978). The ACC/AHA/NASPE recommended guidelines for permanent and temporary implantation of pacemakers in patients with an acute MI and shown in Tables 2 and 3.

REFERENCES

1. Antiarrhythmics Versus Implantable Defibrillators (AVID) Investigators. A comparison of antiarrhythmic-drug therapy with implantable defibrillators in patients resuscitated from near-fatal ventricular arrhythmias. The Antiarrhythmics versus Implantable Defibrillators (AVID) Investigators. N Engl J Med 337:1576–1583, 1997.
2. Antzelevitch C, Brugada P, Borggrefe M, et al. Brugada syndrome: report of the second consensus conference. Heart Rhythm 2:429–440, 2005.
3. Atlee JL. Perioperative cardiac dysrhythmias: diagnosis and management. Anesthesiology 86:1397–1424, 1997.
4. Atrial Fibrillation Investigators. Risk factors for stroke and efficacy of antithrombotic therapy in atrial fibrillation. Analysis of pooled data from five randomized controlled trials. Arch Intern Med 154:1449–1457, 1994.
5. Bardy GH, Lee KL, Mark DB, et al. Amiodarone or an implantable cardioverter-defibrillator for congestive heart failure. N Engl J Med 352:225–237, 2005.
6. Bauernfeind RA, Amat YLF, Dhingra RC, Kehoe R, Wyndham C, Rosen KM. Chronic nonparoxysmal sinus tachycardia in otherwise healthy persons. Ann Intern Med 91:702–710, 1979.
7. Belhassen B, Glick A, Viskin S. Efficacy of quinidine in high-risk patients with Brugada syndrome. Circulation 110:1731–1737, 2004.
8. Blomstrom-Lundqvist C, Scheinman MM, Aliot EM, et al. ACC/AHA/ESC guidelines for the management of patients with supraventricular arrhythmias—executive summary: a report of the American College of Cardiology/American Heart Association Task Force on Practice Guidelines and the European Society of Cardiology Committee for Practice Guidelines (Writing Committee to Develop Guidelines for the Management of Patients With Supraventricular Arrhythmias). Circulation 108:1871–1909, 2003.
9. Brugada P, Brugada J, Mont L, Smeets J, Andries EW. A new approach to the differential diagnosis of a regular tachycardia with a wide QRS complex. Circulation 83:1649–1659, 1991.
10. Campbell RW, Smith RA, Gallagher JJ, Pritchett EL, Wallace AG. Atrial fibrillation in the preexcitation syndrome. Am J Cardiol 40:514–520, 1977.
11. Cardiac Arrhythmia Suppression Trial II Investigators. Effect of the antiarrhythmic agent moricizine on survival after myocardial infarction. N Engl J Med 327:227–233, 1992.
12. Carlsson J, Miketic S, Windeler J, et al. Randomized trial of rate-control versus rhythm-control in persistent atrial fibrillation: the Strategies of Treatment of Atrial Fibrillation (STAF) study. J Am Coll Cardiol 41:1690–1696, 2003.
13. Chen Q, Kirsch GE, Zhang D, et al. Genetic basis and molecular mechanism for idiopathic ventricular fibrillation. Nature 392:293–296, 1998.
14. Chen SA, Tai CT, Yu WC, et al. Right atrial focal atrial fibrillation: electrophysiologic characteristics and radiofrequency catheter ablation. J Cardiovasc Electrophysiol 10:328–335, 1999.
15. Echt DS, Liebson PR, Mitchell LB, et al. Mortality and morbidity in patients receiving encainide, flecainide, or placebo. The Cardiac Arrhythmia Suppression Trial. N Engl J Med 324:781–788, 1991.

16. Fuster V, Ryden LE, Asinger RW, et al. ACC/AHA/ESC guidelines for the management of patients with atrial fibrillation: executive summary. A Report of the American College of Cardiology/ American Heart Association Task Force on Practice Guidelines and the European Society of Cardiology Committee for Practice Guidelines and Policy Conferences (Committee to Develop Guidelines for the Management of Patients With Atrial Fibrillation): developed in Collaboration With the North American Society of Pacing and Electrophysiology. J Am Coll Cardiol 38:1231–1266, 2001.

17. Gage BF, Waterman AD, Shannon W, Boechler M, Rich MW, Radford MJ. Validation of clinical classification schemes for predicting stroke: results from the National Registry of Atrial Fibrillation. Jama 285:2864–2870, 2001.

18. Go AS, Hylek EM, Phillips KA, et al. Prevalence of diagnosed atrial fibrillation in adults: national implications for rhythm management and stroke prevention: the AnTicoagulation and Risk Factors in Atrial Fibrillation (ATRIA) Study. Jama 285:2370–2375, 2001.

19. Goldschlager N, Epstein AE, Naccarelli G, Olshansky B, Singh B. Practical guidelines for clinicians who treat patients with amiodarone. Practice Guidelines Subcommittee, North American Society of Pacing and Electrophysiology. Arch Intern Med 160:1741–1748, 2000.

20. Greenberg H, Case RB, Moss AJ, Brown MW, Carroll ER, Andrews ML. Analysis of mortality events in the Multicenter Automatic Defibrillator Implantation Trial (MADIT-II). J Am Coll Cardiol 43:1459–1465, 2004.

21. Gregoratos G, Cheitlin MD, Conill A, et al. ACC/AHA Guidelines for Implantation of Cardiac Pacemakers and Antiarrhythmia Devices: Executive Summary—a report of the American College of Cardiology/American Heart Association Task Force on Practice Guidelines (Committee on Pacemaker Implantation). Circulation 97:1325–1335, 1998.

22. Grogin HR, Scheinman M. Evaluation and management of patients with polymorphic ventricular tachycardia. Cardiol Clin 11:39–54, 1993.

23. Haissaguerre M, Jais P, Shah DC, et al. Spontaneous initiation of atrial fibrillation by ectopic beats originating in the pulmonary veins. N Engl J Med 339: 659–666, 1998.

24. Hart RG, Pearce LA, McBride R, Rothbart RM, Asinger RW. Factors associated with ischemic stroke during aspirin therapy in atrial fibrillation: analysis of 2012 participants in the SPAF I–III clinical trials. The Stroke Prevention in Atrial Fibrillation (SPAF) Investigators. Stroke 30:1223–1229, 1999.

25. Hindman MC, Wagner GS, Jaro M, et al. The clinical significance of bundle branch block complicating acute myocardial infarction. Indications for temporary and permanent pacemaker insertion. Circulation 58:689–699, 1978.

26. Hohnloser SH, Kuck KH, Dorian P, et al. Prophylactic use of an implantable cardioverter-defibrillator after acute myocardial infarction. N Engl J Med 351: 2481–2488, 2004.

27. Hohnloser SH, Kuck KH, Lilienthal J. Rhythm or rate control in atrial fibrillation—Pharmacological Intervention in Atrial Fibrillation (PIAF): a randomised trial. Lancet 356:1789–1794, 2000.

28. Jackman WM, Wang XZ, Friday KJ, et al. Catheter ablation of accessory atrioventricular pathways (Wolff-Parkinson-White syndrome) by radiofrequency current. N Engl J Med 324:1605–1611, 1991.
29. Jais P, Haissaguerre M, Shah DC, et al. A focal source of atrial fibrillation treated by discrete radiofrequency ablation. Circulation 95:572–576, 1997.
30. Jalife J. Experimental and clinical AF mechanisms: bridging the divide. J Interv Card Electrophysiol 9:85–92, 2003.
31. Kastor J. Arrhythmias. Philadelphia: WB Saunders, 1994.
32. Lee KL, Chun HM, Liem LB, Sung RJ. Effect of adenosine and verapamil in catecholamine-induced accelerated atrioventricular junctional rhythm: insights into the underlying mechanism. Pacing Clin Electrophysiol 22:866–870, 1999.
33. Levine JH, Michael JR, Guarnieri T. Treatment of multifocal atrial tachycardia with verapamil. N Engl J Med 312: 21–25,1985.
34. Manning W, J., Silverman DI, Gordon SPF, Krumholz HM, Douglas PS. Conversion from atrial fibrillation without prolonged anticoagulation with use of transesophageal echocardiography to exclude the presence of atrial thrombi. N Engl J Med 328:750–755, 1993.
35. Marriott HJL. Practical Electrocardiography. Baltimore: Williams & Wilkins, 1988.
36. Mazgalev TN, Tchou PJ. Surface potentials from the region of the atrioventricular node and their relation to dual pathway electrophysiology. Circulation 101:2110–2117, 2000.
37. McCord J, Borzak S. Multifocal atrial tachycardia. Chest 113:203–209, 1998.
38. Moss AJ, Hall WJ, Cannom DS, et al., and Investigators MADIT. Improved survival with an implanted defibrillator in patients with coronary disease at high risk for ventricular arrhythmia. N Engl J Med 335:1933–1940, 1996.
39. Moss AJ, Zareba W, Hall WJ, et al. Prophylactic implantation of a defibrillator in patients with myocardial infarction and reduced ejection fraction. N Engl J Med 346:877–883, 2002.
40. Myerburg RJ, Mitrani R, Interian A, Jr, Castellanos A. Interpretation of outcomes of antiarrhythmic clinical trials: design features and population impact. Circulation 97:1514–1521, 1998.
41. Napolitano C, Priori SG, Schwartz PJ. Torsade de pointes. Mechanisms and management. Drugs 47:51–65, 1994.
42. Priori SG, Aliot E, Blomstrom-Lundqvist C, et al. Task Force on Sudden Cardiac Death of the European Society of Cardiology. Eur Heart J 22:1374–1450, 2001.
43. Rathore SS, Berger AK, Weinfurt KP, et al. Acute myocardial infarction complicated by atrial fibrillation in the elderly: prevalence and outcomes. Circulation 101:969–974, 2000.
44. Roden DM. Torsade de pointes. Clin Cardiol 16:683–686, 1993.
45. Scheinman MM, Huang S. The 1998 NASPE prospective catheter ablation registry. Pacing Clin Electrophysiol 23:1020–1028, 2000.
46. Snow V, Weiss KB, LeFevre M, et al. Management of newly detected atrial fibrillation: a clinical practice guideline from the American Academy of Family Physicians and the American College of Physicians. Ann Intern Med 139: 1009–1017, 2003.

47. Van Gelder IC, Hagens VE, Bosker HA, et al. A comparison of rate control and rhythm control in patients with recurrent persistent atrial fibrillation. N Engl J Med 347:1834–1840, 2002.

48. Wang L, Yao R. Radiofrequency catheter ablation of accessory pathway-mediated tachycardia is a safe and effective long-term therapy. Arch Med Res 34: 394–398, 2003.

49. Wilde AA, Antzelevitch C, Borggrefe M, et al. Proposed diagnostic criteria for the Brugada syndrome. Eur Heart J 23:1648–1654, 2002.

50. Wolf PA, Dawber TR, Thomas HE, Jr, Kannel WB. Epidemiologic assessment of chronic atrial fibrillation and risk of stroke: the Framingham study. Neurology 28:973–977, 1978.

51. Wood MA, Brown-Mahoney C, Kay GN, Ellenbogen KA. Clinical outcomes after ablation and pacing therapy for atrial fibrillation: a meta-analysis. Circulation 101:1138–1144, 2000.

52. Wyse DG, Waldo AL, DiMarco JP, et al. A comparison of rate control and rhythm control in patients with atrial fibrillation. N Engl J Med 347:1825–1833, 2002.

3 Prevention of Bacterial Endocarditis

Bacterial endocarditis, although uncommon, is a life-threatening disease with substantial morbitity and mortality. Endocarditis usually develops in individuals with underlying structural cardiac defects who develop bacteremia with organisms likely to cause endocarditis.

Endocarditis usually occurs after a transient bacteremia seeds either a damaged heart valve or the endocardium near anatomic defects. Although bacteremia is common following many invasive procedures, only certain bacteria commonly cause endocarditis. The risk of endocarditis depends on both the structural cardiac abnormalities and the degree of bacteremia with the procedure, thus so preventive efforts are focused on patients with structural cardiac abnormalities. The individuals at highest risk are those who have prosthetic heart valves, a previous history of endocarditis (even in the absence of other heart disease), complex cyanotic congenital heart disease, or surgically constructed systemic pulmonary shunts or conduits (Steckelberg & Wilson, 1993).

The incidence of endocarditis following most procedures in patients with underlying cardiac disease is low. Professional societies in both the United States and Europe have formulated approaches for endocarditis prophylaxis, weighing the degree to which the patient's underlying condition creates a risk of endocarditis, the risk of bacteremia with the procedure, and the risk–benefit ratio of the prophylactic antimicrobial regimen under consideration (Dajani et al., 1997; Horstkotte et al., 2004). In the United States, the American Heart Association (AHA) guidelines for antibiotic prophylaxis for certain patients undergoing dental, genitourinary (GU), gastrointestinal (GI), and respiratory procedures are the most widely followed (Dajani, 1997).

From: *Current Clinical Practice: Cardiology in Family Practice: A Practical Guide*
By: S. M. Hollenberg and T. Walker © Humana Press Inc., Totowa, NJ

Table 1
Cardiac Conditions and Endocarditis Prophylaxis

Endocarditis prophylaxis recommended

High-risk category

- Prosthetic cardiac valves, including bioprosthetic and homograft valves
- Previous bacterial endocarditis
- Complex cyanotic congential heart disease (e.g., single ventricle states, transposition of the great arteries, tetralogy of Fallot)
- Surgically constructed systemic-pulmonary shunts or conduits

Moderate-risk category

- Congenital cardiac malformations other than those listed in the high-risk and negligible-risk categories
- Acquired valvular dysfunction (e.g., rheumatic heart disease)
- Hypertrophic cardiomyopathy
- Mitral valve prolapse with valvular regurgitation and/or thickened leaflets

Endocarditis prophylaxis not recommended

Negligible-risk category (no greater risk than the general population)

- Isolated secundum atrial septal defect
- Surgical repair of atrial septal defect, ventricular septal defect or patent ductus arteriosus (without residua beyond 6 months)
- Previous coronary artery bypass graft surgery
- Mitral valve prolapse without valvular regurgitation
- Physiologic, functional, or innocent heart murmur
- Previous Kawasaki disease without valvular dysfunction
- Previous rheumatic fever without valvular dysfunction
- Cardiac pacemakers (intravascular and epicardial) and implanted defibrillators

Adapted from Dajani et al. (1997).

The AHA stratifies certain cardiac conditions into high, moderate, and negligible risk for developing bacterial endocarditis. This risk stratification is based on the potential outcome if endocarditis occurs (Dajani et al., 1997). Antibiotic prophylaxis is recommended for all patients in the high and moderate risk groups. Table 1 describes the cardiac conditions associated with each risk category.

Table 2
Dental Procedures and Endocarditis Prophylaxis

Endocarditis prophylaxis recommended

- Dental extractions
- Periodontal procedures, including surgery, scaling, root planing, probing, and recall maintenance
- Dental implant placement and reimplantation of avulsed teeth
- Endodontic instrumentation or surgery only beyond the apex
- Subgingival placement of antibiotic fibers or strips
- Initial placement of orthodontic bands (but not brackets)
- Intraligamentary local anesthetic injections
- Prophylactic cleaning of teeth or implants, where bleeding is anticipated

Endocarditis prophylaxis not recommended

- Restorative dentistry (operative and prosthodontic), with or without retraction cord
- Local anesthetic injections (nonintraligamentary)
- Intracanal endodontic treatment (post-placement and build-up)
- Placement of rubber dams
- Postoperative suture removal
- Placement of removable prosthodontic or orthodontic appliances
- Oral impressions, fluoride treatments, oral radiographs
- Orthodontic appliance adjustment
- Shedding of primary teeth

Adapted from Dajani et al. (1997).

The dental procedures for which antibiotic prophylaxis is recommended are listed in Table 2. The respiratory, GU , and GI procedures for antibiotic prophylaxis recommendations are listed in Table 3. For GI procedures, antibiotic prophylaxis is recommended only for patients in the high-risk category and is considered optional for the moderate-risk category.

Antibiotic therapy should be directed at the most common organism associated with each medical procedures. α-Hemolytic *Streptococci* of the *viridans* group is associated with procedures involving the oral, respiratory, and esophageal mucosa. The AHA now recommends only a single pre-procedure antibiotic dose be given for dental,

Table 3
Other Procedures and Endocarditis Prophylaxis

Endocarditis prophylaxis recommended

    Respiratory tract
- Tonsillectomy and/or adenoidectomy
- Surgical procedures that involve respiratory mucosa
- Rigid bronchoscopy

    Gastrointestinal tract [a]
- Sclerotherapy for esophageal varices
- Esophageal stricture dilation
- Endoscopic retrograde choloangiography with biliary obstruction
- Biliary tract surgery
- Surgical procedures that involve intestinal mucosa

    Genitourinary tract
- Prostatic surgery
- Cystoscopy, urethral dilation

Endocarditis prophylaxis not recommended

    Respiratory tract
- Endotracheal intubation, flexible bronchoscopy with or without biopsy
- Tympanostomy tube insertion

    Gastrointestinal tract
- Transesophageal echocardiography [b]
- Endoscopy with or without biopsy [b]

    Genitourinary tract
- Vaginal hysterectomy or delivery [b]
- Cesarean section in uninfected tissue
- Urethral catheteriztion
- Uterine dilatation and curettage
- Therapeutic abortion
- Sterilization procedures
- Insertion or removal of intrauterine devices

    Other procedures
- Cardiac catheterization, including balloon angioplasty
- Coronary stents and implanted pacemakers and defibrillators
- Incision or biopsy of sugically scrubbed skin
- Circumcision

[a] Prophylaxis recommended for high-risk patients, and optional for moderate-risk.
[b] Prophylaxis optional for high-risk patients.
Adapted from Dajani et al. (1997).

Table 4
Endocarditis Prophylactic Regimens for Dental,
Oral, Respiratory, and Esophageal Procedures

Situation	Agent	Regimen[a]
Standard general prophylaxis	Amoxicilllin	Adults: 2 g; children 50 mg/kg orally 1 h before procedure
Unable to take oral medications	Ampicillin	Adults: 2 g IM or IV; Children 50 mg/kg IM or IV Within 30 min before procedure
Penicillin allergic	Clindamycin or	Adults: 600 mg; children 20 mg/kg orally 1 h before procedure
	Cefadroxil[b] or	Adults 2 g; children 50 mg/kg
	Cephalexin[b] or	Orally 1 h before procedure
	Azithromycin	Adults: 500 mg; children 15 mg/kg Orally 1 h before procedure
Penicillin allergic and unable to take oral medications	Clindamycin or	Adults: 600 mg; children 20 mg/kg IV within 30 min before procedure
	Cefazolin	Adults: 1 g; children 25 mg/kg IM or IV 30 min before procedure

[a] Total pediatric dose should not exceed the adult dose.

[b] Cephalosporins should not be used in patients with an immediate-type hypersensitivity reaction (urticaria, angioedema or anaphylaxis) to penicillins.

Adapted from Dajani et al. (1997).

respiratory, and esphogeal procedures (Dajani et al., 1997). The recommended regimen is 2 g of amoxicillin, given orally pre-procedure, a dose that has prolonged serum levels and inhibitory activity. Erythromycin is no longer recommended for patients with an allergy to penicillin; clindamycin, cephalexin, and cefadroxil or azithromycin should be used (Dajani et al., 1997). *Enterococcus faecalis* has the potential to cause bacterial endocarditis following certain GU and GI procedures. Although bacteremia with Gram-negative bacilli occurs with these procedures, endocarditis occurs only rarely. Therefore, the antibiotic regimen is geared to treating *Enterococcus*. Tables 4 and 5 list the prophylactic antibiotic regimens for all oral, respiratory GI,

Table 5
Endocarditis Prophylactic Regimens
for Genitourinary and Gastrointestinal Procedures[a]

Situation	Agent	Regimen
High-risk patients	Ampicillin plus Gentamicin	Adults: ampicillin 2 g IM or IV, plus gentamicin, 1.5 mg/kg IM or IV (not to 120 mg), giving within 30 min of starting procedure; 6 h later, ampicillin, 1g IM or IV or amoxicillin, 1 g orally[b] Children: ampicillin, 50 mg/kg IM or IV (not to exceed 2.0 g) plus gentamicin,1.5 mg/kg, within 30 min of starting procedure; 6 h later, ampicillin, 25 mg/kg IM or IV or amoxicillin, 25 mg/kg orally[b]
High-risk patients allergic to ampicillin/ amoxicillin	Vancomycin plus gentamicin	Adults: Vancomycin 1 g IV over 1–2 h, plus gentamicin 1.5 mg/kg IV or IM (not to exceed 120 mg). Should be completed within 30 min of starting procedure[b] Children: Vancomycin 20 mg/kg IV over 1–2 h, plus gentamicin 1.5 mg/kg IV or IM; completed within 30 min of starting procedure[b]

(Continued on next page)

and GU procedures. All patients in the high-risk category undergoing a GU or GI procedure should receive parental antibiotics.

It is important to recognize that when endocarditis develops in individuals with underlying cardiac conditions, the severity of the disease and the ensuing morbidity can be variable. No randomized controlled trials in patients have demonstrated definitely that antibiotic prophylaxis provides protection against procedure-induced endocarditis. In this area, as in most of medicine, adaptation of

Table 5 *(Continued)*
Endocarditis Prophylactic Regimens
for Genitourinary and Gastrointestinal Procedures[a]

Situation	Agent	Regimen
Moderate-risk patients	Amoxicillin or ampicillin	Adults: amoxicillin 2 g orally 1 h before procedure, or ampicillin 2 g IM/IV within 30 min of starting procedure Children: amoxicillin 50 mg/kg orally 1 h before procedure, or ampicillin 50 mg/kg IM/IV within 30 min of starting procedure
Moderate-risk patients allergic to ampicillin/ amoxicillin	Vancomycin	Adults: vancomycin 1 g IV over 1–2 h completed within 30 min of starting procedure[b] Children: vancomycin 20 mg/kg IV over 1–2 h; completed with 30 min of starting procedure[b]

[a] Excluding esophageal procedures.
[b] A second dose of vancomycin or gentamicin is not recommended.
Adapted from Dajani et al. (1997).

general guidelines to individual patients is necessary. Prophylaxis is particularly important for individuals in whom endocardial infection is associated with high morbidity and mortality.

REFERENCES

1. Dajani AS, Taubert KA, Wilson W, et al. Prevention of bacterial endocarditis. Recommendations by the American Heart Association. JAMA 277:1794–1801, 1997.
2. Horstkotte D, Follath F, Gutschik E, et al. Guidelines on prevention, diagnosis and treatment of infective endocarditis executive summary; the task force on infective endocarditis of the European society of cardiology. Eur Heart J 25: 267–276, 2004.
3. Steckelberg JM, Wilson WR. Risk factors for infective endocarditis. Infect Dis Clin North Am 7:9–19, 1993.

4   Congestive Heart Failure

DEFINITION AND EPIDEMIOLOGY

Congestive heart failure (CHF) can be defined as the inability of the heart to provide an adequate cardiac output without invoking maladaptive compensatory mechanisms. CHF affects more than 4 million patients in the United States, nearly 2% of the adult population (American Heart Association [AHA], 2004). Some 400,000 patients develop heart failure for the first time every year, and CHF results in 200,000 cardiovascular deaths and 1 million hospital admissions per year in the United States. CHF is now the most common reason for hospitalization in the elderly, and annual costs are estimated at more than $25 billion (AHA, 2004) The incidence of heart failure has been increasing, not only as a result of the aging of the population but also because improved treatment of hypertension and coronary disease is allowing patients to avoid early mortality only to develop heart failure later.

The causes of heart failure are protean, and are listed in Table 1. The predominant causes, however, are ischemia, hypertension, alcoholic cardiomyopathy, myocarditis, and idiopathic cardiomyopathy. Coronary artery disease (CAD) is increasing, both as a primary cause and as a complicating factor.

Heart failure can be broken down into several different classifications: acute versus chronic, left-sided versus right-sided, systolic versus diastolic dysfunction. It is important for the clinician, to distinguish between systolic and diastolic dysfunction, as both the diagnostic work-up and therapeutic sequence differs. Although CHF results most commonly from decreased systolic performance, diastolic dysfunction, defined clinically as cardiogenic pulmonary congestion in the presence of normal systolic performance, is becoming more common as a cause of CHF particularly in the elderly. The

From: *Current Clinical Practice: Cardiology in Family Practice:*
A Practical Guide
By: S. M. Hollenberg and T. Walker © Humana Press Inc., Totowa, NJ

Table 1
Etiologies of Congestive Heart Failure

- Ischemic
- Hypertensive
- Idiopathic
- Valvular
- Peripartum
- Familial
- Metabolic/nutritional
- Toxic
  ◇ Alcoholic
  ◇ Radiation
  ◇ Drug-related (anthracyclines)
  ◇ Heavy metals (cobalt, lead, arsenic)
- Systemic diseases
  ◇ Hypothyroidism
  ◇ Connective tissue disease
  ◇ Diabetes
  ◇ Sarcoidosis
- Infiltrative
  ◇ Amyloidosis
  ◇ Hemochromatosis
- Tachycardia-induced
- Autoimmune

estimated prevalence of diastolic heart failure is 30 to 35% overall, and more than 50% in patients older than 70 (Zile & Brutsaert, 2002).

The severity of chronic heart failure is most commonly delineated using the classification developed by the New York Heart Association (NYHA). This classification divides patients into functional classes depending on the degree of effort needed to elicit symptoms (*see* Table 2). More recently, stages in the evolution of heart failure have been proposed by an American College of Cardiology/AHA task force, to emphasize its progressive nature and to focus on preventive measures and early intervention (*see* Table 3). These stages have been linked to therapeutic approaches (*see* Fig. 1).

Table 2
New York Heart Association
Functional Classification of Heart Failure

Class I:	Symptoms of heart failure only at levels that would limit normal individuals
Class II:	Symptoms of heart failure with ordinary exertion
Class III:	Symptoms of heart failure on less than ordinary exertion
Class IV:	Symptoms of heart failure at rest

Table 3
Stages of Heart Failure

Stage A:	High risk for heart failure, without structural disease or symptoms
Stage B:	Heart disease with asymptomatic left ventricular dysfunction
Stage C:	Prior or current symptoms of heart failure
Stage D:	Advanced heart disease and severely symptomatic or refractory heart failure

PATHOPHYSIOLOGY

Heart failure is a syndrome caused not only by the low cardiac output resulting from compromised systolic performance, but also by the effects of compensatory mechanisms. Myocardial damage from any cause can produce myocardial failure. To compensate for the reduced cardiac output of a failing heart, an elevation in ventricular filling pressure occurs in an attempt to maintain output via the Frank-Starling law. These elevated diastolic filling pressures can compromise subendocardial blood flow and cause or worsen ischemia. With continued low cardiac output, additional compensatory mechanisms come into play, including sympathetic nervous system stimulation, activation of the renin–angiotensin system, and vasopressin secretion. All of these mechanisms lead to sodium and water retention and venoconstriction, increasing both preload

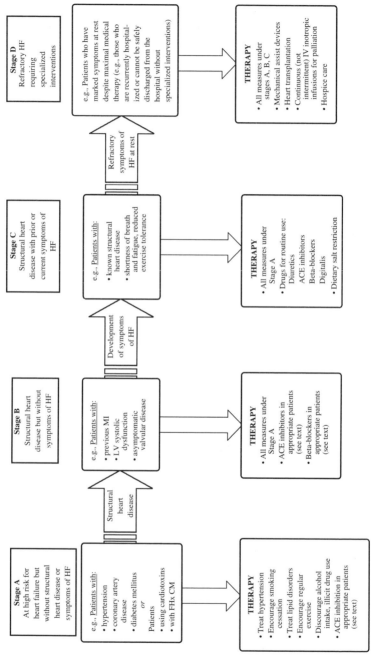

Stage A
At high risk for heart failure but without structural heart disease or symptoms of HF

e.g., Patients with:
• hypertension
• coronary artery disease
• diabetes mellitus
or
Patients
• using cardiotoxins
• with FHx CM

THERAPY
• Treat hypertension
• Encourage smoking cessation
• Treat lipid disorders
• Encourage regular exercise
• Discourage alcohol intake, illicit drug use
• ACE inhibition in appropriate patients (see text)

Structural heart disease

Stage B
Structural heart disease but without symptoms of HF

e.g., Patients with:
• previous MI
• LV systolic dysfunction
• asymptomatic valvular disease

THERAPY
• All measures under Stage A
• ACE inhibitors in appropriate patients (see text)
• Beta-blockers in appropriate patients (see text)

Development of symptoms of HF

Stage C
Structural heart disease with prior or current symptoms of HF

e.g., Patients with:
• known structural heart disease
• shortness of breath and fatigue, reduced exercise tolerance

THERAPY
• All measures under Stage A
• Drugs for routine use:
  Diuretics
  ACE inhibitors
  Beta-blockers
  Digitalis
• Dietary salt restriction

Refractory symptoms of HF at rest

Stage D
Refractory HF requiring specialized interventions

e.g., Patients who have marked symptoms at rest despite maximal medical therapy (e.g., those who are recurrently hospitalized or cannot be safely discharged from the hospital without specialized interventions)

THERAPY
• All measures under stages A, B, C
• Mechanical assist devices
• Heart transplantation
• Continuous (not intermittent) IV inotropic infusions for palliation
• Hospice care

and afterload. These increases in preload and afterload, although initially compensatory, can exacerbate the heart failure, because elevated preload increases pulmonary congestion, and elevated afterload impedes cardiac output.

Recent attention has focused on cardiac remodeling, the process by which ventricular size, shape, and function are regulated by mechanical, neurohormonal, and genetic factors, as a pathophysiological mechanism in heart failure. Remodeling may be physiological and adaptive during normal growth, but excessive remodeling after myocardial infarction (MI), cardiomyopathy, hypertension, or valvular heart disease can be maladaptive (Sutton & Sharpe, 2000). Early local remodeling after MI may expand the infarct zone, but late remodeling, which likely involves neurohormonal mechanisms initiated by hemodynamic stress, involves the left ventricle globally and is associated with dilation that increases over time, distortion of ventricular shape, and hypertrophy of the walls. Failure to normalize increased wall stresses results in progressive dilatation and deterioration in contractile function. Similar processes are operative in other sorts of cardiomyopathy as well. Ventricular remodeling can be considered a primary target for treatment and a reliable surrogate for long-term outcomes (Sutton & Sharpe, 2000).

DIAGNOSIS

The symptoms and signs of CHF relate both to low cardiac output and elevated ventricular filling pressures. Low output produces the symptoms of weakness and fatigue and an ashen appearance, sometimes with mottling. Increased left-sided filling pressures result in symptoms of pulmonary congestion such as dyspnea, cough, orthopnea, and paroxysmal nocturnal dyspnea as well as signs that may include tachycardia, pulmonary rales, a diffuse, enlarged and laterally displaced point of maximal impulse, an S3 and S4 gallop, a murmur of mitral regurgitation. Elevated right-sided preload can lead to symptoms such as anorexia, nausea, and abdominal pain

---

Fig. 1. *(Opposite page)* Stages in the evolution of heart failure and recommended therapy by stage. HF, heart failure; FHx CM, family history of cardiomyopathy; MI, myocardial infarction; LV, left ventricular; ACE, angiotension-converting enzyme; IV, intravenous.

along with signs of systemic congestion such as jugular venous distension, a right-sided S3 gallop, a murmur of tricuspid regurgitation, hepatomegaly, ascites, and peripheral edema.

The presentation of acute heart failure and pulmonary edema can be dramatic, with sudden onset of shortness of breath and tachypnea with use of accessory muscles. Crackles and often wheezing can be heard throughout the lung fields, at times obscuring some of the cardiac auscultatory findings. Hypotension and evidence of peripheral vasoconstriction and hypoperfusion may be present if cardiac output is decreased. The differential diagnosis of cardiac pulmonary edema includes other causes of acute dyspnea such as pulmonary embolism, pneumothorax, and bronchial asthma and causes of non-cardiac pulmonary edema such as aspiration, infection, toxins, or trauma.

Initial evaluation of the patient with pulmonary edema should include an electrocardiogram and chest x-ray. The electrocardiogram may show evidence of myocardial ischemia and can also detect arrhythmias; conduction abnormalities such as arterioventricular (AV) block and bundle branch block may be diagnosed. Q-waves indicative of previous MI or criteria diagnostic of ventricular hypertrophy may provide clues about the substrate for heart failure; atrial enlargement speaks to chronicity of elevated filling pressures. The chest x-ray can demonstrate pulmonary vascular redistribution, with or without bilateral hazy pulmonary infiltrates, classically perihilar, as well as cardiomegaly. Pleural effusions may be identified but are neither sensitive nor specific.

Laboratory evaluation should include baseline serum electrolytes and creatinine, blood glucose to detect underlying diabetes, liver function tests, which may indicate hepatic congestion, and a complete blood count because anemia can exacerbate pre-existing CHF.

Recently, measurement of plasma B-type natriuretic peptide (BNP) has been introduced into t the diagnostic algorithm for CHF. BNP is produced by ventricular myocytes in response to increased wall stress (i.e., increased filling pressures and stretch). Plasma BNP levels are increased in heart failure, and plasma concentration of BNP has been shown to correlate with NYHA functional class. Measurement of BNP has been used to distinguish between heart failure and pulmonary causes of dyspnea. In the Breathing Not Properly study, plasma BNP was measured with a rapid assay in 1586 patients presenting to the emergency room with a chief complaint of dyspnea; 47% were diagnosed with CHF, 49% no CHF, and 5% were felt to have noncardiac dyspnea in the setting of left venricular (LV) dysfunction (Maisel et al., 2002). Plasma BNP greater than 400 pg/mL accurately predicted CHF, whereas levels less than 100 pg/mL indicated non-cardiac dyspnea; values between 100 and 400 pg/mL were less useful (Maisel et al., 2002). Such intermediate values may be the result of CHF but may also represent pre-existing LV dysfunction or right-sided failure. Addition of echocardiography in the acute setting may be especially valuable in patients with intermediate BNP levels (Logeart et al., 2002).

Echocardiography can provide important information about cardiac size and function and should be performed in all patients with new-onset heart failure. Echocardiography is simple, safe, and permits systemic interrogation of cardiac chamber size, LV and right ventricular function, valvular structure and motion, atrial size, and pericardial anatomy. Regional wall motion abnormalities are compatible with CAD, but are not specific for ischemia because they are also seen in 50 to 60% of patients with idiopathic dilated cardiomyopathy. Fibrotic and thinned akinetic areas, however, do indicate previous infarction. Doppler echocardiography can be used to evaluate the severity of mitral and tricuspid regurgitation, and the tricuspid regurgitation velocity can be used to estimate pulmonary artery pressure. In addition, Doppler echocardiography is increasingly used in the diagnosis of diastolic dysfunction.

Patients presenting with heart failure should be assessed for the presence of CAD, and thus stress testing should be considered. Either nuclear or echocardiographic imaging is usually added to increase sensitivity, although both present interpretive pitfalls in patients with severe global ventricular dysfunction. Some patients may be better served by proceeding directly to diagnostic cardiac catheterization. Even in the presence of known coronary atherosclerosis, however, stress testing may be useful to identify viable myocardium if revascularization is under consideration. In patients with severe heart failure, measurement of maximal oxygen uptake with exercise can provide an extremely useful prognostic measure (Hunt et al., 2001).

Cardiac catheterization represents the gold standard for exclusion of significant CAD, and should be considered in most patients with new-onset heart failure, even those with no anginal symptoms, unless co-morbid conditions render the risk prohibitive or would preclude any invasive therapy. In addition to coronary angiography, measurements of cardiac output and filling pressures can be useful both prognostically and therapeutically. In addition, endomyocardial biopsy can be performed in selected cases if an unusual cause of myocarditis is suspected.

THERAPY
Treatment Goals

The goals of CHF therapy are to control symptoms, improve exercise tolerance, prolong life, and where possible, correct the underlying cause. Different therapies can have disparate effects on these goals.

The therapeutic agents can be viewed in the light of the pathophysiological mechanisms of CHF development. Traditionally, these have been considered in hemodynamic terms. Fluid restriction, diuretics, and venodilators decrease cardiac preload. Angiotensin-converting enzyme (ACE) inhibitors, angiotensin receptor blockers (ARBs), and aldosterone antagonists counteract activation of the renin–angiotensin–aldosterone system and reduce afterload as well. Arterial dilators can also reduce afterload. Inotropic agents can improve cardiac pump function and increase output. More recently, effects of therapy on counterproductive neurohormonal activation have received attention. β-Blockers can counteract sympathetic activation and are being used more commonly in heart failure management. The most current approaches, however, take into account the effects of different therapies on ventricular remodeling. Therapies that have been shown to have a beneficial effect on remodeling, such as ACE inhibitors, ARBs, aldosterone antagonists, and β-blockers, reduce mortality and are effective across the whole spectrum of heart failure severity. Mechanical approaches to remodeling, most notably cardiac resynchronization therapy, also appear to be effective.

General Measures

The first order of business in the therapy of new or decompensated CHF is to address the precipitating causes, the most prominent of which are listed in Table 4. Bypass surgery or percutaneous inter-

Table 4
Precipitating Causes of Congestive Heart Failure

- Myocardial ischemia or infarction
- Excess salt or fluid intake
- Noncompliance or inadequate drug regimen
- Renal failure
- Arrhythmias
- Anemia
- Infection
- Fever
- Thytotoxicosis
- Pregnancy
- Pulmonary embolism

vention for cardiac ischemia can improve both symptoms and ventricular performance. Registry data consistently support the notion that in the presence of significant amounts of ischemic yet viable myocardium, revascularization confers a survival benefit (CASS Principal Investigators, 1985). For patients with arrhythmias, either cardioversion or rate control can produce marked improvement.

Patients with acute heart failure should be put at bed rest (which by itself can produce a diuresis), with sodium restriction to less than 2 g per day and fluid restriction in severe cases. Attention should be paid to prophylaxis for deep venous thrombosis.

PHARMACOLOGICAL THERAPY

Diuretics

Diuretics cause renal sodium and water loss, decreasing preload and thus pulmonary and systemic congestion. For inpatient treatment of decompensated heart failure, loop diuretics such as furosemide are usually chosen initially because of their rapid onset and are given as intravenous boluses. When used for patients who present with pulmonary edema, most of the rapid effect of furosemide is attributable to venodilation.

If there is no response to a bolus dose of a loop diuretic, the dose is titrated to achieve desired effect, usually by doubling the dose.

Loop diuretics enter the glomerulus primarily by tubular secretion in the proximal tubule and so exhibit a threshold effect. Once the effective dose has been determined, the degree of diuresis is usually adjusted by changing the frequency of diuretic administration. If intermittent bolus doses of loop diuretics are ineffective or are poorly tolerated due to large fluid shifts and consequent hypotension, continuous infusion may be preferable (Dormans et al.,1996). Alternatively, another diuretic with a different mechanism of action, such as metolazone or chlorthiazide may be added.

Use of diuretics can lead to significant hypokalemia or hypomagnesemia, which can predispose the patient to arrhythmias. Careful addition of a potassium-sparing diuretic can be considered in some settings.

Nitrates

Nitrates are still first-line agents for the symptomatic relief of angina pectoris and when MI is complicated by CHF. Given the high incidence of CAD in patients with CHF, use of nitrates to reduce preload is often desirable. In severely decompensated CHF, intravenous nitroglycerin is preferred because of questionable absorption of oral and transdermal preparations and for ease of titration. Intravenous nitroglycerin should be started at 5 µg per minute and increased in increments of 5 µg per minute every 3 to 5 minutes as needed for symptomatic relief. The major adverse effects of nitrates are hypotension and headache.

Long-term therapy with oral nitrates alone does not impact ventricular remodeling and thus, In the absence of ongoing ischemia, is not usually a first-line choice. When combined with hydralazine, however, salutary effects on outcome have been demonstrated, first in the Valsartan in Heart Failure trial (V-HeFT) (Cohn et al., 1986), and more recently in the African-American Heart Failure trial (Taylor, 2004). These trials are described in the section on hydralazine.

Angiotensin-Converting Enzyme Inhibitors

ACE inhibitors inhibit conversion of angiotensin I to angiotensin II and also inhibit breakdown of bradykinin. Both of these actions produce vasodilation, the latter through bradykinin-induced nitric oxide (NO) production, but the increased inhibition of ventricular remodeling seen with ACE inhibitors compared to other vasodilators speaks to the potential for involvement of other mechanisms. Local renin–angiotensin systems, both intracardiac and intravascular, contribute to myocardial hypertrophy and remodeling, and their inhibition by ACE inhibitors may explain part of their beneficial effects (Dzau et al., 2001). ACE inhibitors also modulate sympathetic nervous system activity, and increased NO production may exert direct beneficial effects on cardiac myocytes.

ACE inhibitors improve hemodynamics, functional capacity, and survival in patients across the spectrum of severity of chronic CHF and also after MI. The Cooperative North Scandanavian Enalapril Survival Study (CONSENSUS) group compared enalapril to placebo in 253 patients with advanced heart failure (NYHA class III or IV) and showed a 40% reduction in 6-month mortality; this benefit was sustained, with a risk reduction averaged over the 10-year duration of the trial of 30% (CONSENSUS Trial Study Group, 1987). The Studies of Left Ventricular Dysfunction (SOLVD) treatment trial compared enalapril with placebo in 2569 patients with symptomatic heart failure (NYHA class II to III) and showed a 16% mortality reduction (SOLVD Investigators, 1991). Moreover, ACE inhibitors also prevented the development of CHF in patients with asymptomatic LV dysfunction in the SOLVD prevention trial (SOLVD Investigators, 1992).

ACE inhibitors also improve the outcome in patients with asymptomatic LV dysfunction or overt heart failure after an acute MI. In the Survival and Ventricular Enlargement (SAVE) trial, 2231 asymptomatic patients with an ejection fraction (EF) less than 40% were randomly assigned to either captopril or placebo. Captopril decreased mortality by 19% at 42 months, and also decreased hospitalization for heart failure and, interestingly, recurrent MI (Pfeffer et al., 1992). The latter effect may have been the result of improvement in endothelial function. The Acute Infarction Ramipril Efficacy (AIRE) trial compared ramipril with placebo in 2006 patients with clinical heart failure and showed a 27% reduction in mortality at 15 months (AIRE Study Investigators, 1993). The survival benefit was maintained long-term in both trials.

Patients should be started on low doses and titrated upward to the range demonstrated beneficial in clinical trials (captopril 50 mg three times daily, enalapril 20 mg twice daily, or lisinopril 40 mg once daily). Side effects of ACE inhibitors include cough, renal failure (usually occurs in the setting of renal artery stenosis), hyperkalemia, and angioedema.

Angiotensin Receptor Blockers

An alternative approach to inhibiting the effects of angiotensin II is use of agents that block the angiotensin II receptor (ARBs). Because these agents do not increase bradykinin, the incidence of some side effects, such as cough and angioedema, is greatly reduced. The hemodynamic effects of ARBs have been shown in a number of trials to be similar to those of ACE inhibitors. Trials comparing ACE inhibitors with ARBs in patients with heart failure have suggested similar mortality reductions (Pitt et al., 2000). Nonetheless, the number of heart failure patients treated with ARBs and followed for mortality is still relatively small compared with ACE inhibitors, and so ARBs are usually reserved for patients who cannot tolerate ACE inhibitors, however, ARBs are a good alternative.

The recent recognition that angiotensin II is produced by pathways other than ACE has provided a rationale for using ACE inhibitors and ARBs in combination. This approach was tested in the recent V-HeFT, in which valsartan or placebo was added to usual therapy in patients with heart failure (Cohn & Tononi, 2001). Although mortality was unchanged, a combined endpoint of mortality and hospital admission for CHF was reduced with valsartan. Subset analysis of this trial yielded the provocative finding that although valsartan improved mortality in patients on ACE inhibitors but not β-blockers, and also those on β-blockers but not ACE inhibitors, when valsartan was added as triple therapy on top of both ACE inhibitors and β-blockers, mortaltiy was increased (Cohn & Tononi, 2001). Other trials, however, have not shown adverse effects of triple combination therapy. In VALIANT, which compared valsartan, captopril, and the combination of the two in patients with acute MI and CHF, an adverse effect of the combination of ARBs, ACE inhibitors, and β-blockers was not seen (Pfeffer et al., 2003). Increased mortaltiy was also not observed when the ARB candesartan was added to ACE inhibitors and β-blockers in heart failure patients CHARM-Added trial (McMurray et al., 2003).

Aldosterone Antagonists

Although aldosterone is predominantly known for its role in regulation of renal sodium and potassium excretion, its neurohumoral effects are gaining increasing recognition. Aldosterone inhibition impacts ventricular remodeling as well. The Randomized Aldactone Evaluation Study (RALES) randomized 1653 patients with NYHA class III and IV heart failure to spironolactone or placebo, and found a reduction in 24-month mortality from 46 to 35% (relative risk [RR] 30%, p < 0.001) (Pitt et al.,1999). Hyperkalemia was uncommon, and the main side effect was gynecomastia. The recently reported EPHESUS trial randomized 6632 patients with LV dysfunction after MI to eplerenone or placebo, and found a 15% reduction in mortality (RR 0.85, confidence interval [CI] 0.75–0.96, p < 0.01). In this trial, hyperkalemia was noted in 5.5% of the eplerenone group compared with 3.9% of the placebo group (p < 0.01), but interestingly, hypokalemia was reduced, from 13.1 to 8.4%.

It should be noted that the doses of aldosterone antagonists used in these heart failure trials were well below those used for diuresis. Nonetheless, careful attention to serum potassium levels is warranted when using these agents for any indication.

β-*Blockers*

Symptomatic heart failure results in activation of neurohumoral mechanisms, including the sympathetic nervous system, which initially support the performance of the failing heart. Long-term activation of the sympathetic nervous system, however, exerts deleterious effects. Circulating catecholamine levels correlate with survival in these patients (Cohn et al., 1984). Sympathetic activation can increase ventricular volumes and pressure by causing peripheral vasoconstriction and by impairing sodium excretion by the kidneys and can also provoke arrhythmias. Chronic stimulation of β-receptors reduces the responsiveness to β-adrenergic agonists due to downregulation and desensitization of the β-receptor and its coupled signaling pathways, and β-blockade can upregulate adrenergic receptor density, restoring inotropic and chronotropic responsiveness (Hunt et al., 2001). Catecholamines induce oxidative stress in cardiac myocytes, potentially leading to programmed cell death, a process counteracted by β-blockers (Lohse et al., 2003). β-Blockers also reduce the circulating level of vasoconstrictors and mitigate their effects, decreasing afterload. Perhaps most importantly, catecholamines promote deleterious ventricular remodeling, and β-blockers can decrease LV end-systolic and end-diastolic volume (Hunt et al., 2001). Thus, although perhaps counterintuitive on hemodynamic grounds, there is now compelling evidence that β-blockers are beneficial not only for patients with acute MI complicated by heart failure but also with CHF from all causes (Hunt et al., 2001).

β-Blockers have now been evaluated in more than 10,000 patients with heart failure and systolic dysfunction. This collective experience indicates that long-term treatment with β-blockers can relieve symptoms, improve ventricular performance, and reduce both mortality and the need for hospitalization. Three different agents have been shown to decrease mortality in patients with NYHA class II and III heart failure: metoprolol XL (Metoprolol CR/XL Randomised Intervention Trial in Congestive Heart Failure Investigators, 1999), bisoprolol (CIBIS-II Investigators, 1999), and carvedilol (Packer et al., 2001). Recent studies with carvedilol suggest that the benefits extend to patients with class IV heart failure (Krum et al., 2003). These benefits of β-blockers are seen in patients with or without CAD and in patients with or without diabetes, and are also observed in patients already taking ACE inhibitors.

Initiation of β-blockers, however, can be problematic during the acute phase of heart failure, as they can depress contractility. When given for heart failure indications *per se*, β-blockers should be introduced when the patient is in a well-compensated and euvolemic state, typically in the ambulatory setting and at low doses. Patients who experience an exacerbation of heart failure while on maintenance β-blocker therapy, particularly at a higher dose, present a previously rare dilemma that is becoming more common. No controlled observations are available to guide therapy, so current practice remains largely at the discretion of individual clinicians. Discontinuing β-blockers, or decreasing their dose, may expose myocardial β-receptors to endogenous catecholamines, and may result in a brief increase in contractility. On the other hand, slow titration of β-blockers will need to begin anew after resolution of acute CHF. It is usually best to attempt to resolve acute episodes of heart failure by diuresis and adjustment of other medications while holding β-blocker doses constant, and to halve the dose if heart failure persists.

Hydralazine

Hydralazine reduces afterload by directly relaxing smooth muscle. Its effects are almost exclusively confined to the arterial bed. In normal subjects, the hypotensive actions of hydralazine provoke a marked reflex tachycardia, but this response is often blunted in with heart failure.

Hydralazine is effective in increasing cardiac output in heart failure. Hydralazine in combination with oral nitrates was the first therapy shown to improve mortality in CHF when given, reducing mortality in patients with class III and IV heart failure in the V-HeFT trial (Cohn et al., 1986). Enalapril was shown to be superior to this combination (Cohn et al., 1991). In addition, oral hydralazine must be given four times a day, and prolonged administration is attended by the development of a lupus-like syndrome in up to 20% of patients, and so hydralazine has usually been reserved for ACE-intolerant patients.

Recently, a fixed dose of both isosorbide dinitrate and hydralazine that is given twice daily was tested in blacks with class III and IV heart failure, a subgroup previously noted to have a favorable response to this therapy and that may not respond as well to ACE inhibition (Taylor et al., 2004). Hydralazine and nitrates improved mortality, heart failure hospitalization, and quality of life (Taylor et al., 2004).

Nesiritide

Nesiritide is a recombinant form of human B-type natriuretic peptide (BNP). BNP assays have been used in the diagnosis of heart failure as described earlier, but when infused intravenously, nesiritide is a vasodilator that also has a natriuretic effect. In patients with heart failure, intravenous nesiritide has been shown to increase stroke volume and cardiac output and to decrease right atrial and pulmonary capillary wedge pressure (PCWP). In the Vasodilation in the Management of Acute Congestive Heart Failure (VMAC) trial, 489 patients, including 246 who underwent pulmonary artery catheterization, were randomly assigned to nesiritide, intravenous nitroglycerin, or placebo for 3 hours, followed nesiritide or intravenous nitroglycerin for 24 hours (VMAC Investigators, 2002). Nesiritide decreased the mean PCWP significantly more than either intravenous nitroglycerin or placebo at 3 hours (5.8 versus 3.8 and 2.0 mmHg) and significantly more than nitroglycerin at 24 hours (8.2 versus 6.3 mmHg). Symptoms of dyspnea were compared with placebo, but not significant compared to intravenous nitroglycerin (VMAC Investigators, 2002). Although nesiritide is natriuretic, it has not been shown to improve either glomerular filtration rate or renal plasma flow (Wang et al., 2004). Studies showing improved outcomes with nesiritide are not yet available. Hypotension is the most common side effect.

Digoxin

Digitalis, which has been used to treat heart failure for more than 200 years, works by inhibiting Na, K-dependent ATPase activity, causing intracellular sodium accumulation and increasing intracellular calcium via the sodium–calcium exchange system. Digoxin improves myocardial contractility and increases cardiac output, but its inotropic effects are mild in comparison to catecholamines. The effect of digoxin on patient survival was definitively addressed in the Digoxin Investigators' Group trial, a study of 6800 patients with symptomatic CHF and systolic dysfunction (Digoxin Investigators Group, 1997) There was no difference in survival between the digoxin and placebo groups, but did decrease in hospitalization for heart failure significantly (Digoxin Investigators Group, 1997). Thus, apart from its use as an antiarrhythmic agent, digoxin is recommended in patients with systolic dysfunction and symptomatic heart failure despite therapy with diuretics, ACE inhibitors, and β-blockers.

Inotropic Agents

In severe decompensated heart failure, inotropic support may be initiated. Dobutamine is a selective β_1-adrenergic receptor agonist that can improve myocardial contractility and increase cardiac output. Dobutamine is the initial inotropic agent of choice in patients with decompensated acute heart failure and adequate systolic blood pressure. Dobutamine has a rapid onset of action and a plasma half-life is 2 to 3 minutes; infusion is usually initiated at 5 μg/kg per minute and then titrated. Tolerance to the effect of dobutamine may develop after 48 to 72 hours, possibly due to downregulation of adrenergic receptors. Dobutamine has the potential to exacerbate hypotension in some patients, and can precipitate tachyarrhythmias.

Milrinone is a phosphodiesterase inhibitor milrinone with both positive inotropic and vasodilatory actions. Because milrinone does not stimulate adrenergic receptors directly, it may be effective when added to catecholamines or when β-adrenergic receptors have been downregulated. Compared with catecholamines, phosphodiesterase inhibitors have fewer chronotropic and arrhythmogenic effects.

Although clearly useful to improve hemodynamics in the acute setting, controversy has arisen regarding use of inotropic agents (other than digoxin) as outpatient maintenance therapy for chronic heart failure. Concerns have included exacerbation of arrhythmic complications, either by induction of myocardial ischemia or by independent pathways, and perpetuation of neurohumoral activation that might accelerate the progression of myocardial damage. Milrinone was recently examined in a prospective manner in the Outcomes of a Prospective Trial of Intravenous Milrinone for Exacerbations of Chronic Heart Failure (OPTIME-CHF) trial in order to determine whether its use could reduce hospitalization time following an acute heart failure exacerbation. Although these observations did not demonstrate any advantage for patients treated with milrinone, patients whom the investigators felt "needed" acute inotropic support were not included in the trial, thereby biasing the enrollment toward a less severely afflicted cohort. Therefore, the utilization of such agents today remains at the discretion of the clinician. The proof that these agents have beneficial effects on hard clinical endpoints remains elusive, but their hemodynamic effects are attractive for treating decompensated patients.

Inotropic infusions need to be titrated carefully in patients with ischemic heart disease to maximize coronary perfusion pressure with the least possible increase in myocardial oxygen demand. Invasive hemodynamic monitoring can be extremely useful to allow for optimization of therapy in these unstable patients, because clinical estimates of filling pressure can be unreliable, and because changes in myocardial performance and compliance and therapeutic interventions can change cardiac output and filling pressures precipitously. Optimization of filling pressures and serial measurements of cardiac output (and other parameters, such as mixed venous oxygen saturation) allow for titration of inotropes and vasopressors to the minimum dosage required to achieve the chosen therapeutic goals, thus minimizing the increases in myocardial oxygen demand and arrhythmogenic potential.

Arrhythmias

Arrhythmias are common in patients with heart failure. Nonsustained ventricular tachycardia (VT) may occur in as many as 50% of patients, and complex ventricular depolarizations in as many as 80%.

Forty to 50% of deaths are sudden, and many of these deaths are attributable to arrhythmias.

The mortality benefits of some of the standard therapies for heart failure, particularly β-blockers, may be attributable in part to anti-arrhythmic properties. Specific antiarrhytmic agents, however, have not proven very effective for the prevention of sudden death in patients with heart failure (Antiarrhythmics Versus Implantable Defibrillators [AVID] Investigators, 1997), and so attention has focused on identifying patients who would benefit from implanation of an implantable cardiac defibrillator (ICD).

Implantation of ICDs as secondary prevention in survivors of sudden cardiac death or patients with hemodynamically significant sustained ventricular tachycardias has been well demonstrated to improve survival in clinical trials (AVID Investigators, 1997); virtually all had of the patients enrolled had LV dysfunction, and about half had clinical heart failure.

ICDs are effective as primary prevention in selected heart failure patients as well. The Multicenter Automatic Defibrillator Implantation (MADIT) I and Multicenter Unsustained Tachycardia (MUSST) trials showed a mortality benefit with ICD in patients with LV dysfunction (EF <35–40%) and nonsustained VT in whom sustained VT was inducible at electrophysiological study (Buxton et al., 1999; Moss et al.,1996). The MADIT II trial showed a mortality benefit with ICD in a trial which the entry criterion was simply an ejection fraction less than 30% (Moss et al., 2002). Most of the patients in these trials had ischemic cardiomyopathy. More recently, the Sudden Cardiac Death in Heart Failure Trial (SCD-HeFT) compared ICD implantation to amiodarone in patients with heart failure resulting from either an ischemic or nonischemic cardiomyopathy (EF <35%), and found a mortality benefit with ICD in both groups (Bardy et al., 2005).

Cardiac Resynchronization

Left bundle branch block or other conduction system abnormalities can cause dyssynchronous ventricular contraction. Such dyssynchrony causes abnormal septal motion, decreasing contractile performance and myocardial efficiency, reduces diastolic filling times, and can increase the duration and degree of mitral regurgitation. The goal of cardiac resynchronization therapy (CRT) is to pace the left and right ventricles to restore physiologic AV timing and contraction synchrony. This is accomplished by placing the standard leads in the right atrium and right ventricle and also placing a special lead through the coronary sinus to enable pacing of the lateral aspect of the left ventricle.

CRT, by optimizing the coordination of contraction, improves LV contractile function, stroke volume, and cardiac output, with decreased pulmonary capillary wedge pressures (PCWPs). This improved performance is associated with either no increase or a decrease in myocardial oxygen consumption, thus increasing myocardial efficiency. Most importantly, biventricular (BiV) pacing is associated with reverse ventricular remodeling. In the Multicenter InSync Randomized Clinical Evaluation (MIRACLE) trial, BiV pacing produced significant decreases in LV end-systolic and end-diastolic dimensions, a significant reduction in mitral regurgitation jet area, and a reduction in LV mass, all signs of reverse remodeling (Abraham et al., 2002). CRT also improved exercise capacity, functional class, and quality of life in this trial (Abraham et al., 2002).

Studies of outcomes after CRT are beginning to emerge (Abraham et al., 2002). The Comparison of Medical Therapy, Pacing, and Defibrillation in Heart Failure (COMPANION) trial compared optimal medical therapy with CRT with and without an ICD in 1520 patients with NYHA class III–IV heart failure and an LVEF less than 35% (Bristow et al., 2004). The primary endpoint, a combination of all-cause mortality and hospitalization, was reduced in both the CRT alone and the CRT plus ICD arm compared with medical therapy (Bristow et al., 2004). The reduction in the secondary endpoint of all-cause mortality alone was significant only in the CRT plus ICD arm compared with medical therapy. In the recently reported Cardiac Resynchronization-Heart Failure (CARE-HF) trial, CRT reduced the interventricular mechanical delay, ventricular volume, and mitral regurgitation, increased EF, improved symptoms and quality of life, and reduced both death and the combined endpoint of death and hospitalization compared with medical therapy (Cleland et al., 2005).

Overview

The goals of heart failure therapy are to reduce symptoms, improve exercise tolerance, and increase survival. Although these are all worthy goals, thus far only therapies that impact ventricular remod-

Table 5
Remodeling and Survival by Drug Class

Established therapy	Remodeling effects	Survival effects
ACE-I	Benefit	Benefit
ARB	Benefit (+ACE better)	Benefit (+ACE better)
Aldosterone	Benefit	Benefit
β-blocker	Benefit	Benefit
Diuretic	No benefit	No benefit
Digoxin	No benefit	No benefit
Other therapies	*Remodeling effects*	*Survival effects*
Endothelin antagonists	No benefit	No benefit
TNF-α	No benefit	No benefit
Inotropes	Adverse	Adverse

ACE, angiotensin-converting enzyme; ARB, angiotensin receptor blocker; TNF, tumor necrosis factor.

eling have been shown to influence mortality (*see* Table 5). Therapies that either prevent or reverse remodeling also tend to be effective across the spectrum of heart failure therapy. Thus, for long-term therapy, the aim is to put patients on the therapies that have been demonstrated in clinical trials to improve mortality, and to titrate the doses of those therapies to the levels achieved in the trials.

DIASTOLIC HEART FAILURE
Definition

There is growing recognition that a sizable number of patients with heart failure do not have a significant abnormality of systolic performance. Diastolic heart failure is a clinical syndrome characterized by the signs and symptoms of heart failure and a preserved EF.

Virtually all patients with diastolic heart failure have a measurable abnormality in ventricular diastolic performance (Zile & Brutsaert, 2002). Nonetheless, the term *diastolic dysfunction* has the potential to cause confusion. Strictly speaking, unequivocal documentation of abnormal diastolic function would require demonstration that the ventricular end-diastolic pressure volume curve is shifted upward, a task that requires simultaneous assessment of both pressure and volume across a wide range of values. What is more commonly present is evidence of elevated end-diastolic pressures or increased diastolic stiffness, a situation that may result from either a shifted compliance curve or from increased LV end-diastolic volume. Because the compensatory response to significant systolic dysfunction usually entails increased end-diastolic volume, it follows that virtually all patients with systolic dysfunction have diastolic dysfunction as well. Diastolic heart failure denotes patients with diastolic dysfunction in the absence of significant systolic dysfunction. Whether documentation of diastolic dysfunction is strictly necessary remains a bit controversial (Zile & Brutsaert, 2002).

Epidemiology

Diastolic heart failure is estimated to account for up to one-third of cases of CHF, with the proportion increasing to almost 50% in the elderly. Thus, diastolic heart failure is becoming more common as the population ages.

The most common causes of diastolic heart failure are hypertension and ischemic heart disease, although other less common etiologies include hypertrophic and restrictive cardiomyopathies and some valvular abnormalities, most prominently aortic stenosis.

Although the prognosis is less ominous for patients with diastolic than systolic heart failure (annual mortality 5–8% compared with 10–15%), mortality exceeds that of age-matched controls (Zile & Brutsaert, 2002). Morbidity is high as well, with similar symptoms and re-admission rates (approaching 50% at 1 year) compared to systolic failure.

Etiology and Diagnosis

Diastolic function has a number of subtleties, and its analysis can become quite complex. Nonetheless, early diastole is the period of ventricular relaxation, and ventricular filling is most important later on. Ventricular relaxation has both active and passive components. The active component is dependent on calcium removal from the myofilaments and cytoplasm, and is energy-dependent. Thus, active relaxation can be impaired by myocardial ischemia. The passive component of relaxation consists of elastic recoil of structural proteins compressed during systole. Chamber filling is reflected in the diastolic pressure-volume relation.

There are a variety of measures, both invasive and noninvasive, for the assessment of diastolic function. Each measurement indexes slightly different features, and none by itself embodies all of the relevant information. By taking several measures together, however, the picture becomes clearer.

Echocardiography is the most useful method for assessment of ventricular function in the clinical setting (Nishimura et al.,1997). First, it provides a measure of systolic performance, allowing for distinction of systolic from diastolic heart failure. Doppler echocardiography of mitral inflow patterns generates measures of early (E velocity) and late (A, corresponding to atrial contraction) filling velocities. In normal heart, the E wave is greater than the A wave. As diastolic dysfunction develops, the E wave decreases (and deceleration time increases) and the A wave increases ("E to A reversal"). With severe diastolic dysfunction, left atrial pressure increases markedly and the E wave becomes much larger than the A wave (with a very short deceleration time), the "restrictive pattern." In between the first and last stages of diastolic dysfunction, there is a pattern known as "pseudonormalization," in which the E and A waves appear normal, but left atrial pressure is increased. Thus, relying only on these patterns and E and A velocities has the potential to generate some confusion. A number of newer and more specific echocardiographic measures are coming into clinical use, including pulmonary and hepatic vein velocities. The most promising is tissue Doppler imaging of the mitral annulus, which moves away from the apex with ventricular filling. The ratio of mitral inflow velocity to mitral annular velocity (E/E′) increases with higher filling pressures; a value greater than 15 is specific for a pulmonary artery occlusion pressure greater than 20 mmHg (Dujardin et al.,1998).

Management

The initial step in treating patients with diastolic heart failure is to reduce pulmonary congestion by decreasing LV volume. Maintaining synchronous atrial contraction is an important adjunct. Treatment of the underlying disease process is of clear importance as well. Blood pressure control should be optimized in hypertensive patients. If ischemia is the inciting cause, then appropriate diagnostic and therapeutic measures should be pursued.

There have been few randomized trials in patients with diastolic heart failure. The largest of these is the CHARM-Preserved trial, which randomized 3023 patients with CHF and EF greater than 40% to the ARB candesartan or placebo (Yusuf et al., 2003). The primary outcome, cardiovascular death or hospitalization for CHF, did not differ between groups (22 versus 24%, hazard ratio 0.89, CI 0.77–1.03, $p = 0.12$), and death was equivalent, but rates of admission were lower with candesartan (Yusuf et al., 2003).

Tachycardia is poorly tolerated in patients with diastolic heart failure, particularly those with the potential for ischemia because myocardial oxygen demand is increased and diastolic filling times are shortened. Thus, β-blockers and calcium channel blockers with negative chronotropic effects can increase exercise tolerance and provide symptomatic improvement. Stroke volumes in patients with diastolic heart failure are generally subnormal, because despite preserved EF, LV cavity size is small (Andrew, 2003). Doses should be individualized with the goal of blunting the tachycardic response to stress and exercise without unduly decreasing resting heart rate and cardiac output.

REFERENCES

1. Abraham WT, Fisher WG, Smith AL, et al. Cardiac resynchronization in chronic heart failure. N Engl J Med 346:1845–1853, 2002.
2. Acute Infarction Ramipril Efficacy (AIRE) Study Investigators. Effect of ramipril on mortality and morbidity of survivors of acute myocardial infarction with clinical evidence of heart failure. Lancet 342:821–828, 1993.
3. American Heart Association. Heart Disease and Stroke Statistics 2004 Update. Dallas, TX: American Heart Association, 2004.
4. Andrew P. Diastolic heart failure demystified. Chest 124:744–753, 2003.
5. Antiarrhythmics Versus Implantable Defibrillators (AVID) Investigators. A comparison of antiarrhythmic-drug therapy with implantable defibrillators in patients resuscitated from near-fatal ventricular arrhythmias. The Antiarrhythmics versus Implantable Defibrillators (AVID) Investigators. N Engl J Med 337:1576–1583, 1997.
6. Bardy GH, Lee KL, Mark DB, et al. Amiodarone or an implantable cardioverter-defibrillator for congestive heart failure. N Engl J Med 352:225–237, 2005.
7. Bristow MR, Saxon LA, Boehmer J, et al. Cardiac-resynchronization therapy with or without an implantable defibrillator in advanced chronic heart failure. N Engl J Med 350:2140–2150, 2004.
8. Buxton AE, Lee KL, Fisher JD, Josephson ME, Prystowsky EN, Hafley G. A randomized study of the prevention of sudden death in patients with coronary

artery disease. Multicenter Unsustained Tachycardia Trial Investigators. N Engl J Med 341:1882–1890, 1999.

9. CASS Principal Investigators. A randomized trial of coronary artery bypass surgery. Survival of patients with a low ejection fraction. N Eng J Med 312:1665–1671, 1985.

10. CIBIS-II Investigators. The Cardiac Insufficiency Bisoprolol Study II (CIBIS-II): a randomised trial. Lancet 353:9–13, 1999.

11. Cleland JG, Daubert JC, Erdmann E, et al. The effect of cardiac resynchronization on morbidity and mortality in heart failure. N Engl J Med, 352: 1539–1549, 2005.

12. Cohn JN, Archibald DG, Ziesche S, et al. Effect of vasodilator therapy on mortality in chronic congestive heart failure. Results of a Veterans Administration cooperative study. N Engl J Med 314:1547–1552, 1986.

13. Cohn JN, Johnson G, Ziesche S, et al. A comparison of enalapril with hydralazine-isosorbide dinitrate in the treatment of chronic congestive heart failure. N Engl J Med 325:303–310, 1991.

14. Cohn JN, Levine TB, Olivari MT, et al. Plasma norepinephrine as a guide to prognosis in patients with chronic congestive heart failure. N Engl J Med 311: 819–823, 1984.

15. Cohn JN Tognoni G. A randomized trial of the angiotensin-receptor blocker valsartan in chronic heart failure. N Engl J Med 345:1667–1675., 2001.

16. CONSENSUS Trial Study Group. Effects of enalapril on mortality in severe congestive heart failure. Results of the Cooperative North Scandanavian Enalapril Survival Study (CONSENSUS). N Engl J Med 316:1429–1435, 1987.

17. Digoxin Investigators Group. The effect of digoxin on mortality and morbidity in patients with heart failure. N Engl J Med 336:525–533, 1997.

18. Dormans TP, van Meyel JJ, Gerlag PG, Tan Y, Russel FG, Smits P. Diuretic efficacy of high dose furosemide in severe heart failure: bolus injection versus continuous infusion. J Am Coll Cardiol 28:376–382, 1996.

19. Dujardin KS, Tei C, Yeo TC, Hodge DO, Rossi A, Seward JB. Prognostic value of a Doppler index combining systolic and diastolic performance in idiopathic-dilated cardiomyopathy. Am J Cardiol 82:1071–1076, 1998.

20. Dzau VJ, Bernstein K, Celermajer D, et al. The relevance of tissue angiotensin-converting enzyme: manifestations in mechanistic and endpoint data. Am J Cardiol 88:1L–20L, 2001.

21. Hunt SA, Baker DW, Chin MH, et al. ACC/AHA Guidelines for the Evaluation and Management of Chronic Heart Failure in the Adult: Executive Summary. Circulation 104:2996–3007, 2001.

22. Krum H, Roecker EB, Mohacsi P, et al. Effects of initiating carvedilol in patients with severe chronic heart failure: results from the COPERNICUS Study. JAMA 289:712–718, 2003.

23. Logeart D, Saudubray C, Beyne P, et al. Comparative value of Doppler echocardiography and B-type natriuretic peptide assay in the etiologic diagnosis of acute dyspnea. J Am Coll Cardiol 40:1794–1800, 2002.

24. Lohse MJ, Engelhardt S, Eschenhagen T. What is the role of beta-adrenergic signaling in heart failure? Circ Res 93:896–906, 2003.

25. Maisel AS, Krishnaswamy P, Nowak RM, et al. Rapid measurement of B-type natriuretic peptide in the emergency diagnosis of heart failure. N Engl J Med 347:161–167, 2002.

26. McMurray JJ, Ostergren J, Swedberg K, et al. Effects of candesartan in patients with chronic heart failure and reduced left-ventricular systolic function taking angiotensin-converting-enzyme inhibitors: the CHARM-Added trial. Lancet 362:767–771, 2003.

27. Metoprolol CR/XL Randomised Intervention Trial in Congestive Heart Failure Investigators. Effect of metoprolol CR/XL in chronic heart failure: Metoprolol CR/XL Randomised Intervention Trial in Congestive Heart Failure (MERIT-HF). Lancet 353:2001–2007, 1999.

28. Moss AJ, Hall WJ, Cannom DS, et al., and Investigators MADIT. Improved survival with an implanted defibrillator in patients with coronary disease at high risk for ventricular arrhythmia. New England Journal of Medicine 335: 1933–1940, 1996.

29. Moss AJ, Zareba W, Hall WJ, et al. Prophylactic implantation of a defibrillator in patients with myocardial infarction and reduced ejection fraction. N Engl J Med 346:877–883, 2002.

30. Nishimura RA, Tajik AJ. Evaluation of diastolic filling of left ventricle in health and disease: Doppler echocardiography is the clinician's Rosetta Stone. J Am Coll Cardiol 30:8–18, 1997.

31. Packer M, Coats AJ, Fowler MB, et al. Effect of carvedilol on survival in severe chronic heart failure. N Engl J Med 344:1651–1658, 2001.

32. Pfeffer MA, Braunwald E, Moye LA, et al., and Investigators. S. Effect of captopril on mortality and morbidity in patients with left ventricular dysfunction after myocardial infarction. Results of the Survival and Ventricular Enlargement Trial. New England Journal of Medicine 327:669–677, 1992.

33. Pfeffer MA, McMurray JJ, Velazquez EJ, et al. Valsartan, captopril, or both in myocardial infarction complicated by heart failure, left ventricular dysfunction, or both. N Engl J Med 349:1893–1906, 2003.

34. Pitt B, Poole-Wilson PA, Segal R, et al. Effect of losartan compared with captopril on mortality in patients with symptomatic heart failure: randomised trial—the Losartan Heart Failure Survival Study ELITE II. Lancet 355:1582–1587, 2000.

35. Pitt B, Zannad F, Remme WJ, et al., and Randomized Aldactone Evaluation Study Investigators. The effect of spironolactone on morbidity and mortality in patients with severe heart failure. N Engl J Med 341:709–717, 1999.

36. SOLVD Investigators. Effect of enalapril on mortality and the development of heart failure in asymptomatic patients with reduced left ventricular ejection fractions. N Engl J Med 327:685–691, 1992.

37. SOLVD Investigators. Effect of enalapril on survival in patients with reduced left ventricular ejection fractions and congestive heart failure. N Engl J Med 325:293–302, 1991.

38. Sutton MG, Sharpe N. Left ventricular remodeling after myocardial infarction: pathophysiology and therapy. Circulation 101:2981–2988, 2000.

39. Taylor AL, Ziesche S, Yancy C, et al. Combination of isosorbide dinitrate and hydralazine in blacks with heart failure. N Engl J Med 351:2049–2057, 2004.

40. VMAC Investigators. Intravenous nesiritide vs nitroglycerin for treatment of decompensated congestive heart failure: a randomized controlled trial. JAMA 287:1531–1540, 2002.
41. Wang DJ, Dowling TC, Meadows Det al. Nesiritide does not improve renal function in patients with chronic heart failure and worsening serum creatinine. Circulation 110:1620–1625, 2004.
42. Yusuf S, Pfeffer MA, Swedberg K, et al. Effects of candesartan in patients with chronic heart failure and preserved left-ventricular ejection fraction: the CHARM-Preserved Trial. Lancet 362:777–781, 2003.
43. Zile MR, Brutsaert DL. New concepts in diastolic dysfunction and diastolic heart failure: Part I: diagnosis, prognosis, and measurements of diastolic function. Part II: causal mechanisms and treatment. Circulation 105:1387–1393, 1503–1508, 2002.

5   Hyperlipidemia

INTRODUCTION

Cardiovascular disease (CVD) is the leading cause of death in the United States for both men and women. Although the precise number of people with elevated lipids depends on the definition chosen, it is clear that hyperlipidemia is one of the most important modifiable risk factors for coronary heart disease in the United States (Expert Panel on Detection Evaluation and Treatment of High Blood Cholesterol in Adults, 2001).

Lipids are transported in lipoproteins, which are complex compounds that contain a nonpolar core of esterified cholesterol and triglyceride covered by a polar surface layer made up of apolipoproteins, phospholipids, and free cholesterol. The major plasma lipoproteins—chylomicrons, very low-density lipoproteins (VLDL), low-density lipoproteins (LDL), and high-density lipoproteins (HDL) are distinguished by lipid content, size, density, electrophoretic mobility, and surface apoproteins. In hyperlipidemia, circulating levels of lipids or lipoproteins are abnormal because of genetic and environmental conditions that alter the production, breakdown, or clearance of plasma lipoproteins from the circulation.

The National Cholesterol Education Program (NCEP) Adult Treatment Panel (ATP) issues guidelines for the detection, evaluation, and treatment of high blood cholesterol in adults. The latest version published in 2001 (ATP III) focused on more aggressive treatment, better identification of patients at risk for developing coronary artery disease (CAD), defining new levels at which low HDL becomes a major heart disease risk factor, therapeutic lifestyle changes to prevent CAD, increased identification on a constellation of heart disease risk factors known as metabolic syndrome, and increased attention on the treatment of high triglycerides (Expert Panel on Detection Evaluation and Treatment of High Blood Cholesterol in Adults, 2001). The

From: *Current Clinical Practice: Cardiology in Family Practice:*
A Practical Guide
By: S. M. Hollenberg and T. Walker © Humana Press Inc., Totowa, NJ

Table 1
Classification of LDL, HDL, and Total Cholesterol

LDL		Total cholesterol		HDL	
<100	Optimal	<200	Desirable	<40	Low
100–129	Near optimal	200–239	Borderline high	>40	High
130–159	Borderline high	>240	High		
160–189	High				
>190	Very high				

LDL, low-density lipoprotein; HDL, high-density lipoprotein.

NCEP approach discusses screening for hyperlipidemia, and then calibrates the intensity of lipid-lowering efforts to the degree of cardiovascular risk. ATP II focused on intensifying lipid-lowering therapy in patients with established coronary heart disease. ATP III affirms the importance of such efforts, but also stresses primary prevention in patients with multiple cardiac risk factors.

Screening

The NCEP recommends screening every 5 years for all adults over the age of 20 (Expert Panel on Detection Evaluation and Treatment of High Blood Cholesterol in Adults, 2001). A fasting lipid profile should contain total cholesterol, LDL, HDL, and triglycerides. If any of these values are abnormal and before initiating drug therapy, the ATP III recommends that all patients be screened for secondary causes of dyslipidemia. These secondary causes include diabetes, hypothyroidism, obstructive liver disease, chronic kidney disease, and drugs that might affect the cholesterol, LDL, and HDL levels. Table 1 lists the ATP III classification of LDL, HDL, and total cholesterol.

RISK CATEGORIES

A key principle underpinning the ATP III guidelines is that the intensity of lipid-lowering therapy should be adjusted to the individual's absolute risk for coronary heart disease (CHD). Both short- (≤10-year) and long-term (>10-year) risk is taken into consideration. Risk assessment is carried out according to Framingham risk scoring, which derives from analysis of the long-term cross-sectional Framingham study (Tables 2 and 3). The risk factors included in the Framingham calculation of 10-year risk are age, total

Table 2
Estimate of 10-Year Risk for Men and Women

Age	Points		Age	Points	
	Men	Women		Men	Women
20–34	–9	–7	55–59	8	8
35–39	–4	–3	60–69	10	10
40–44	0	0	65–69	11	12
45–49	3	3	70–74	12	14
50–54	6	6	75–79	13	16

Total cholesterol	Age									
	20–39		40–49		50–59		60–69		70–79	
	M	W	M	W	M	W	M	W	M	W
<160	0	0	0	0	0	0	0	0	0	0
160–199	4	4	3	3	2	2	1	1	0	1
200–239	7	8	5	6	3	4	1	2	0	1
240–279	9	11	6	8	4	5	2	3	1	2
>280	11	13	8	10	5	7	3	4	1	2

Smoking	Age									
	20–39		40–49		50–59		60–69		70–79	
	M	W	M	W	M	W	M	W	M	W
Nonsmoker	0	0	0	0	0	0	0	0	0	0
Smoker	8	9	5	7	3	4	1	2	1	1

HDL	Points (men and women)
>60	–1
50–59	0
40–49	1
<40	2

Systolic blood pressure	Untreated		Treated	
	M	W	M	W
<120	0	0	0	0
120–129	0	1	1	3
130–139	1	2	2	4
140–159	1	3	2	5
>160	2	4	3	6

Adapted from the Expert Panel on Detection, Evaluation, and Treatment of High Blood Cholesterol in Adults (2001).

Table 3
Calculation of a Patient's 10-Year Risk

Total points	10-Year risk (%) M	W	Total points	10-Year risk (%) M	W
<0	<1	<1	15	0	3
0–4	1	<1	16	25	4
5–6	2	<1	17	30	5
7	3	<1	18	>30	6
8	4	<1	19	>30	8
9	5	1	20	>30	11
10	6	1	21	>30	14
11	8	1	22	>30	17
12	0	1	23	>30	22
13	12	2	24	>30	27
14	16	2	>25	>30	>30

Adapted from the Expert Panel on Detection, Evaluation, and Treatment of High Blood Cholesterol in Adults (2001).

cholesterol, HDL cholesterol, systolic blood pressure, treatment for hypertension, and cigarette smoking (Wilson et al., 1998).

High Risk

The criteria for high risk include patients with CHD or CHD risk equivalents. Risk equivalents carry the same risk as CAD and include diabetes mellitus, peripheral vascular disease, carotid artery disease, abdominal aortic aneurysm, and a calculated 10-year risk of a coronary event greater than 20% by the Framingham risk score (Tables 2 and 3). There is a very high-risk category based on the presence of established CVD and any one of the following: (a) major risk factors (especially diabetes), (b) severe and poorly controlled risk factors (e.g., smoking), (c) multiple risk factors of the metabolic syndrome (triglycerides >200 mg/dL, non-HDL >130 mg/dL, HDL < 40 mg/dL), or (d) patients with acute coronary syndrome (ACS).

Moderately High Risk

Patients are categorized as moderately high risk if they have two or more risk factors and a 10-year risk for a coronary event between 10 and 20% based on the Framingham risk score (Tables 2 and 3).

Moderate Risk

Patients are considered at moderate risk if they have two or more risk factors and a 10-year risk for a coronary event of less than 10% based on the Framingham risk score (Tables 2 and 3).

Low Risk

Patients are categorized as low risk if they have zero or one risk factor.

Risk Factors

Risk factors include smoking, hypertension (blood pressure >140/90 mmHg or on antihypertensive medications), low HDL (<40 mg/dL), family history of first-degree relatives with premature CHD (in males, age <55; in females, age <65), age (men >45 years old; women >55 years old). An HDL cholesterol of more than 60 mg/dL counts as a negative risk factor, and one risk factor should be removed from the total count (Expert Panel on Detection Evaluation and Treatment of High Blood Cholesterol in Adults, 2001).

METABOLIC SYNDROME

Metabolic syndrome is a constellation of risk factors that increase a person's risk of developing diabetes and CVD. Three of the following criteria are required to meet the diagnosis of metabolic syndrome:

1. Abdominal obesity.
2. Elevated triglyceride level (>150 mg/dL).
3. A low HDL level(<40mg/dL in males or <50 mg/dL in females).
4. High fasting glucose level (>110 mg/dL).
5. High blood pressure (>130/85 mmHg).

TRIGLYCERIDE LEVEL

A recent meta-analysis found that hypertriglyceridemia was an independent risk factor for CHD (Austin et al., 1998). ATP III classified serum triglycerides into the following categories:

- Normal: less than 150 mg/dL
- Borderline-high: 150–199 mg/dL
- High 200–499 mg/dL
- Very high: more than 500 mg/dL (Expert Panel on Detection Evaluation and Treatment of High Blood Cholesterol in Adults, 2001).

Another approach that takes hypertriglyceridemia into account is to calculate non-HDL cholesterol.

Therapy

Therapeutic lifestyle changes (TLC) should be initiated for all patients with an LDL that is above goal. TLC includes reduction in saturated fat (to <7% of total calories), cholesterol intake (to <200 mg per day), weight reduction, and increased physical activity. Patients in the high or moderately high-risk category with lifestyle risk factors are candidates for TLC regardless of their LDL levels. Lifestyle-related risk factors include obesity, elevated triglycerides, low HDL, metabolic syndrome, or physical inactivity.

For patients at high risk, the goal LDL is less than 100 mg/dL. When the LDL is more than 100 mg/dL, a lipid-lowering drug plus TLC should be initiated. ATP III also advised that therapy be intensified to achieve at least a 30–40% reduction in LDL (Expert Panel on Detection Evaluation and Treatment of High Blood Cholesterol in Adults, 2001). If a high-risk patient has elevated triglycerides or low HDL, then a fibrate or nicotinic acid should be considered as an additional agent.

For moderately high-risk patients, the goal LDL is less than 130 mg/dL. Lipid-lowering medication should be initiated if the LDL is greater than 130 mg/dL.

For patients at moderate risk, the goal LDL should be less than 130 mg/dL. If the LDL is greater than 130 mg/dL, then TLC should be initiated. Lipid-lowering medications should be started if the LDL is greater than 160 mg/dL. A therapeutic option is to lower the LDL to less than 100 mg/dL, and to initiate drug therapy in patients with a baseline LDL of 100–129 mg/dL (Grundy et al., 2004). As with high-risk patients, a reduction of 30–40% is recommended (Grundy et al., 2004).

For patients at low risk, the goal LDL is less than 160 mg/dL. TLC should be initiated at an LDL greater than 160 mg/dL. Drug therapy is optional, if after adequate TLC, the LDL cholesterol is between 160 and 189 mg/dL. If the LDL is higher than 190 mg/dL, then drug therapy should be initiated.

Elevated triglycerides can occur in patients who are obese, patients who have diabetes, hypothyroidism, nephrotic syndrome, and other familial genetic disorders; or those on estrogen replacement therapy or β-blocker or immunosuppressive therapy. Achievement of the LDL goal is particularly important for patients with a triglyceride level higher than 150 mg/dL. Weight loss and increased physical activity should be emphasized. For patients with high triglyceride levels, the ATP III recommends that the non-HDL (total cholesterol-HDL cholesterol) be at target with use of a lipid-lowering drug, nicotinic acid, or fibrate (Expert Panel on Detection Evaluation and Treatment of High Blood Cholesterol in Adults, 2001). In patients with very high triglycerides, a low-fat diet, weight loss, increased physical activity, and a triglyceride-lowering drug should be initiated.

Metabolic syndrome is a risk factor for developing CVD and type 2 diabetes. Lifestyle modification (e.g., weight reduction, increased physical activity, diet) and cardiovascular risk reduction (lipid lowering, blood pressure and glycemic control) are crucial in preventive efforts for these patients.

Since the publication of ATP III in 2001, the results of several major clinical trials of statin therapy have reinforced the need for changes in these guidelines, and even the modifications issued in 2003 (Grundy et al., 2004) are probably out of date. A review of the most recent findings from clinical trials provides the most current data and helps identify emerging trends.

The Heart Prevention Study (HPS) evaluated 20,536 adults at high risk for developing CHD and randomized patients to either 40 mg of simvastatin per day or placebo (Heart Protection Study Collaborative Group, 2002). The treatment group had reductions in all-cause mortality (13%), major vascular events (24%), coronary death (18%), nonfatal myocardial infarction (MI) or coronary death (27%), fatal or nonfatal stroke (25%), and coronary revascularization (24%)%) (Heart Protection Study Collaborative Group, 2002). A subgroup analysis showed similar reductions in risk regardless of LDL levels.

The Prospective Study of Pravastatin in the Elderly at Risk (PROSPER) studied 5804 patients over 70 years of age at high risk for developing CVD (Shepherd et al., 2002). Patients were randomized to either 40 mg of pravastatin daily or placebo, and the treatment group showed a reduction of 15% in the composite end-point of coronary death, nonfatal MI, or fatal or nonfatal stroke (Shepherd et al., 2002).

A substudy of the Antihypertension and Lipid Lowering Treatment to Prevent Heart Attack Trial–Lipid-Lowering Trial (ALLHAT-LLT) compared pravastatin to usual care in 10,355 older, hypertensive patients with hypercholesterolemia and at least one cardiovascular risk factor (ALLHAT Investigators, 2002). The study population included substantial proportions of women (49%), African Americans (38%), and Hispanics (23%), and the mean age was 66. Although the all-cause mortality and CHD event rates were similar in both groups, there was substantial crossover in the usual care group to statin therapy, and African Americans showed a significant reduction in risk (ALLHAT Investigators, 2002).

The Anglo-Scandinavian Cardiac Outcomes Trial (ASCOT) randomized 19,342 hypertensive patients young and old (ages 40–79 years) with three cardiovascular risk factors to 10 mg of atorvastatin versus placebo (Sever et al., 2003). The baseline LDL (132 mg/dL) was reduced by 29% in the treatment group. The primary endpoint was cardiac death and nonfatal MI, and trial was stopped early because of a significant reduction (36%) in this combined endpoint. A significant reduction in total coronary events (29%), total cardiovascular events (21%), and stroke (48%) was found, but the reduction in all-cause mortality (13%) did not reach statistical significance in the relatively short follow-up time reported in the manuscript (Sever et al., 2003).

The target lipid levels were the subject of the Pravastatin or Atorvastatin Evaluation and Infection Therapy–Thrombolysis in Myocardial Infarction 22 Trial (PROVE-IT TIMI-22) study of 4162 patients comparing a high-dose statin (atorvastatin 80 mg daily) versus a modest dose (pravastatin 40 mg daily) in patients who had been hospitalized for an ACS (Cannon et al., 2004). The results showed that high-dose statins produced a larger reduction in LDL cholesterol, 62 mg/dL versus 95 mg/dL ($p < 0.001$), and this led to a 16% reduction in the primary composite end point of all-cause mortality, MI, unstable angina requiring hospitalization, revascularization, or stroke at a mean follow-up of 24 months. In a *post hoc* analysis of this study, there were improved clinical outcomes of patients with low levels of serum C-reactive protein (<2 mg/L) after initiation of therapy, irrespective of the achieved LDL cholesterol level (Ridker et al., 2005).

These new clinical trials have given us a better understanding of the benefits of aggressive lipid lowering for patients in the high-risk

Table 4
Drugs Affecting Lipoprotein Metabolism

Drug class	Lipid/lipoprotein	Effects
HMG-CoA reductase inhibitors (statins)	LDL	Decrease by 18–55%
	HDL	Increase by 5–15%
	TG	Decrease by 7–30%
Bile acid sequestrants	LDL	Decrease by 15–30%
	HDL	Increase by 3–5%
	TG	No change or increase
Nicotinic acid	LDL	Decrease by 5–25%
	HDL	Increase by 15–35%
	TG	Decrease by 20–50%
Fibric acids	LDL	Decrease by 5–20% (may be increased in patients with high TG)
	HDL	Increase by 10–20%
	TG	Decrease by 20–50%

Adapted from the Expert Panel on Detection, Evaluation, and Treatment of High Blood Cholesterol in Adults (2001). HMG-CoA, hydroxy-methyl-glutaryl-coenzyme A; LDL, low-density lipoprotein; HDL, high-density lipoprotein; TG, triglycerides.

groups and the elderly. They have also stressed the important of initiating therapy in the hospital, which not only has demonstrable benefits in terms of clinical events, but greatly increases compliance (Fonarow et al., 2001). In 2004, the ATP III issued updated, more aggressive guidelines based on these clinical trials (Grundy et al., 2004). The recommendation of a target LDL of 100 mg/dL may not hold up, however, given evidence of improved outcomes when LDL is lowered to 70 mg/dL (Cannon et al., 2004; LaRosa et al., 2005).

Lipid-Lowering Drugs

Table 4 lists the lipid-lowering agents, and expected changes in the lipid profile. Hydroxy-methyl-glutaryl-coenzyme A (HMG-CoA) inhibitors, or statins, inhibit the rate-limiting step in cholesterol biosynthesis. Statin therapy is the first-line drug of choice for all patients with hypercholesterolemia and has been proven to reduce cardiovascular events. Side effects include increased liver enzymes and myalgias. Approximately 1% of patients taking statins will experience an increase in liver enzymes more than three times normal, usually within 3 months of starting therapy. These changes are usually transient and rarely associated with clinical consequences, but some patients will have continued elevation, and occasional patients will develop symptoms of hepatitis, necessitating discontinuation of the statin. Both symptoms and elevated liver enzymes usually resolve with removal of the drug. Myalgia is the other major side effect of statins, and also occurs less than 1% of the time. The risk of myopathy is increased with concomitant use of several drugs, including fibrates, nicotinic acid, erythromycin, and cyclosporin. Changing from one statin to another sometimes results in resolution of myalgia, but some patients need to stop therapy. Occasional patients experience myopathy severe enough to produce myositis (muscle pain with fever and weakness) or even rhabdomyolysis.

Fibric acid derivatives (fibrates) increase fatty acid oxidation and lipoprotein lipase activity, resulting in lower triglyceride levels and higher HDL levels. Fibrates are generally well tolerated. Side effects from fibrates include cholelithiasis, gastrointestinal upset, and myopathies, which are more frequent in patients taking a fibrate and a statin.

Nicotinic acid (niacin) inhibits the mobilization of free fatty acids from peripheral tissues to the liver, decreasing hepatic VLDL synthesis and release. Niacin is the most effective agent to raise HDL levels. Side effects with nicotinic acid are common but usually mild, and include flushing, nausea, itching, paresthesias, insulin resistance, and hyperuricemia. Pretreatment with aspirin 30 minutes prior to ingestion helps reduce the flushing. Hepatotoxicity is the most serious adverse effect, and liver functions should be monitored.

Bile-acid sequestrants interrupt enterohepatic circulation of bile acids, which increases the conversion of cholesterol into bile acids in the liver as a result of loss of feedback inhibition. Bile-acid sequestrant, either along or in combination with statins can reduce LDL levels. Side effects of these drugs include, nausea, bloating, cramping, increased liver enzymes, and decreased absorption of drugs such as digoxin, warfin, and fat-soluble vitamins. Bile-acid sequestrants can increase triglyceride levels and are therefore not used as monotherapy for patients with hypertriglyceridemia.

Ezetimibe is a new cholesterol-lowering agent that blocks the absorption of cholesterol by the small intestine. Ezetimibe can lower cholesterol when used along with statins, but is usually employed in combination with them. The combination of low doses of ezetimibe and statins can be as effective in lowering LDL as high doses of statins alone (Davidson et al., 2002). Ezetimibe is generally well tolerated and has little interaction with other medications.

REFERENCES

1. ALLHAT Investigators. Major outcomes in moderately hypercholester-olemic, hypertensive patients randomized to pravastatin vs usual care: The Antihypertensive and Lipid-Lowering Treatment to Prevent Heart Attack Trial (ALLHAT-LLT). JAMA 288:2998–3007, 2002.
2. Austin MA, Hokanson JE, Edwards KL. Hypertriglyceridemia as a cardiovas-cular risk factor. Am J Cardiol 81:7B–12B, 1998.
3. Cannon CP, Braunwald E, McCabe CH, et al. Intensive versus moderate lipid lowering with statins after acute coronary syndromes. N Engl J Med 350:1495–1504, 2004.
4. Davidson MH, McGarry T, Bettis R, et al. Ezetimibe coadministered with simvastatin in patients with primary hypercholesterolemia. J Am Coll Cardiol 40:2125–2134, 2002.
5. Expert Panel on Detection Evaluation and Treatment of High Blood Choles-terol in Adults. Executive Summary of the third report of the National Choles-terol Education Program (NCEP) expert panel on detection, evalution, and treatment of high blood cholesterol in adults (Adult Treatment Panel III). JAMA 285:2486–2496, 2001.
6. Fonarow GC, Gawlinski A, Moughrabi S, Tillisch JH. Improved treatment of coronary heart disease by implementation of a Cardiac Hospitalization Athero-sclerosis Management Program (CHAMP). Am J Cardiol 87:819–822, 2001.
7. Grundy SM, Cleeman JI, Merz CN, et al. Implications of recent clinical trials for the National Cholesterol Education Program Adult Treatment Panel III Guidelines. J Am Coll Cardiol 44:720–732, 2004.
8. Heart Protection Study Collaborative Group. MRC/BHF Heart Protection Study of cholesterol lowering with simvastatin in 20,536 high-risk individuals: a randomised placebo-controlled trial. Lancet 360:7–22, 2002.
9. LaRosa JC, Grundy SM, Waters DD, et al. Intensive lipid lowering with atorvastatin in patients with stable coronary disease. N Engl J Med 352:1425–1435, 2005.
10. Ridker PM, Cannon CP, Morrow D, et al. C-reactive protein levels and out-comes after statin therapy. N Engl J Med 352:20–28, 2005.
11. Sever PS, Dahlof B, Poulter NR, et al. Prevention of coronary and stroke events with atorvastatin in hypertensive patients who have average or lower-than-

average cholesterol concentrations, in the Anglo-Scandinavian Cardiac Outcomes Trial—Lipid Lowering Arm (ASCOT-LLA): a multicentre randomised controlled trial. Lancet 361:1149–1158, 2003.

12. Shepherd J, Blauw GJ, Murphy MB, et al. Pravastatin in elderly individuals at risk of vascular disease (PROSPER): a randomised controlled trial. Lancet 360:1623–1630, 2002.

13. Wilson PW, D'Agostino RB, Levy D, Belanger AM, Silbershatz H, Kannel WB. Prediction of coronary heart disease using risk factor categories. Circulation 97:1837–1847, 1998.

ings on two different occasions. Prehypertension is not intended to indicate disease category, but rather to identify individuals at high risk of developing hypertension, and to target those individuals for preventive efforts (Chobanian, 2003).

Once the patient is determined to be prehypertensive or hypertensive, evaluation is begun for lifestyle and cardiovascular risk factors, secondary causes of high BP and the presence or absence of target organ damage (Chobanian, 2003). The physician should inquire about cigarette smoking, obesity, family history of CVD, alcohol use, physical activity, and other cardiovascular risk factors (hyperlipidemia, diabetes, sedentary lifestyle). Factors that may point to secondary causes of hypertension, particularly use of prescription or nonprescription drugs, merit scrutiny.

A compete physical examination and diagnostic test should be performed to evaluate for signs of end-organ damage and secondary causes of hypertension. BP should be obtained in both arms. A funduscopic exam should be performed to evaluate for papilledema, retinal hemorrhages or exudates, arteriovenous (AV) nicking or arteriolar narrowing. The cardiothoracic examination should include evaluation of jugular venous pressure, heart size, and auscultation for murmurs, gallops, rales, or rhonchi. The carotid, subclavian, femoral, and renal arteries should be auscultated for bruits. The abdomen should be examined for renal masses or aortic or renal artery bruits, the extremities examined for edema, and peripheral pulses palpated. The diagnostic work-up should include an electrocardiogram (ECG), complete blood count (CBC), chemistry panel with attention to electrolytes, blood urea nitrogen, creatinine, glucose, and calcium, urinalysis, and a fasting lipid profile. Echocardiography is more sensitive for left ventricular (LV) hypertrophy than ECG, and identifies patients with a worse prognosis (Devereux, 1993).

THERAPY

Lifestyle modifications have shown to reduce BP and CVD complications. Lifestyle modifications include weight reduction, the Dietary Approaches to Stop Hypertension (DASH) diet (rich in fruits, vegetables, grains, low fat dairy products, fish, and poultry), limiting sodium to less than 2.4 g per day, regular exercise, and moderation of alcohol intake. The DASH trial showed that adherence to the DASH diet lowered systolic BP (SBP) by 5.5 mmHg and diastolic BP (DBP) by 3.0 mmHg more than a control diet without weight reduction or a restricted sodium diet (Appel, 1997). This trial also showed a reduction in BP of normotensive subjects participating in the study (Appel, 1997). The DASH-Sodium trial added low salt intake (3 g per day compared with the average intake of 9 g in developed countries) to the DASH diet, and SBP was reduced by 7.1 mmHg (Sacks, 2001). Lifestyle modification is thus encouraged for patients classified as normotensive (BP >120/80) but *recommended* for prehypertensive and hypertensive patients. All patients should be counseled on the benefits of smoking cessation.

The approach recommended in JNC VII bases therapeutic recommendations on both the degree of hypertension and the underlying risk of CVD. Patients are divided into those with uncomplicated hypertension and those with high-risk conditions, which are termed *compelling indications* for the use of other antihypertensive drug classes (*see* Table 2).

For hypertensive patients without compelling indications, thiazide diuretics should be the first drug of choice (Chobanian, 2003). This recommendation was based largely on the outcome of the Antihypertensive and Lipid-Lowering Treatment to Prevent Heart Attack Trial (ALLHAT), which randomized, 33,357 participants over age 55 with hypertension and at least one other coronary risk factor to chlorthalidone, amlodipine, or lisinopril (an arm with doxazosin was stopped early owing to adverse outcomes). The primary endpoint was a combination of death and nonfatal MI. At a mean follow-up of 4.9 years, there was no difference in either the primary outcome or all-cause mortality among treatments (ALLHAT Collaborative Research Group, 2002) Compared directly, diuretics were equivalent to amlodipine, but superior to lisinopril, although this may have been due to improved BP control with chlorthalidone (ALLHAT Collaborative Research Group, 2002). Angiotensin-converting enzyme (ACE) inhibitors, angiotension II blockers, calcium channel blockers (CCBs) and β-blockers may need to be added to maintain the BP at goal. If the BP is 20/10 mmHg above goal, then two drugs may be required as initial therapy, with one being a thiazide diuretic (Chobanian, 2003). Care should be taken to avoid postural hypotension in the elderly and in patients with autonomic dysfunction.

Table 2
Classification and Management of Blood Pressure (BP) for Adults

BP classification	Systoloc BP (mmHg)	Diastolic BP (mmHg)	Lifestyle modification	Drug therapy without compelling indications	Drug therapy with compelling indications
Normal	>120 and	>80	Encourage	None	Drugs for the compelling indications.
Prehypertension	120–139 or	80–89	Yes	None	Drugs for the compelling indications. Other antihypertensive drugs (diurectic, ACEI, ARB, BB, CCB) as needed.
Stage 1 hypertension	140–159 or	90–99	Yes	Thiazide-type diuretics for most. May consider ACEI, ARB, BB, CCB, or combination.	Drugs for the compelling indications. Other antihypertensive drugs (diurectic, ACEI, ARB, BB, CCB) as needed.
Stage 2 hypertension	<160 or	<100	Yes	Two-drug combination for most (usually thiazide-type diuretic and ACEI or ARB or BB or CCB).	Drugs for the compelling indications. Other antihypertensive drugs (diurectic, ACEI, ARB, BB, CCB) as needed.

ACEI, angiotensin-converting enzyme inhibitor; ARB, angiotensin receptor blocker; BB, β-blocker; CCB, calcium channel blocker.

Adapted from Chobanian (2003).

121

COMPELLING INDICATIONS

For patients with hypertension and compelling indications, the treatment recommendations have been modified (Table 3). Hypertension and ischemic coronary disease are the most common causes of heart failure. Patients with heart failure must restrict their sodium and fluid intake. In these patients, BP control is achieved with agents proven to improve outcomes in heart failure. Loop diuretics are used to relieve the symptoms of heart failure. ACE inhibitors improve mortality in patients with systolic dysfunction (CONSENSUS Trial Study Group, 1987; SOLVD Investigators, 1991, 1992). Angiotensin receptor blockers (ARBs) have also been shown to reduce heart failure mortality (Cohn, 2001; Pitt, 2000). β-Blockers relieve symptoms, improve ventricular performance, and reduce both mortality and the need for hospitalization in heart failure patients (CIBIS-II Investigators, 1999; Metoprolol CR/XL Randomised Intervention Trial in Congestive Heart Failure Investigators, 1999; Packer, 1996). The aldosterone antagonist spironolactone reduced the morbidity and death in patients with severe heart failure, albeit at nondiuretic doses (Pitt, 1999). Along similar lines, after MI, survival benefits have been shown with β-blockers (Dargie, 2001; International Collaborative Study Group, 1984), ACE inhibitors (Pfeffer, 1992), and the aldosterone antagonist eplerenone (Pitt, 2003).

The target BP for diabetics is now less than 130/80 and to achieve this level of control, more than one drug is usually required (Chobanian, 2003). Diuretics, β-blockers, ACE inhibitors, ARBs, and CCBs can all be used in the treatment of hypertension in diabetics. Both ACE inhibitors (Jafar, 2003) and ARBs (Brenner, 2001) have been shown to reduce the rate of progression of renal disease in diabetes.

BP should be aggressively treated in patients with chronic kidney disease. As with diabetes, the target BP is less than 130/80, with SBP as the target for antihypertensive therapy. Patients usually require more than three drugs to control their hypertension. ACE inhibitors have been the shown to be renal protective (GISEN [Gruppo Italiano di Studi Epidemiologici in Nefrologia] Group, 1997; Ruggenenti, 1999).

BP lowering is also beneficial for stroke prevention. According to The PROGRESS Trial, using a combination ACE inhibitor and

Table 3
Guideline Basis for Compelling Indications for Individual Drug Classes

Compelling indications	Recommended drugs					
	Diuretic	*BB*	*ACEI*	*ARB*	*CCB*	*Aldo Antag*
Heart failure	X	X	X	X		X
Post-MI		X	X			X
High coronary disease risk	X	X	X		X	
Diabetes	X	X	X	X	X	
Chronic kidney disease			X	X		
Recurrent stroke prevention	X		X			

ACEI, angiotensin-converting enzyme inhibitor; ARB, angiotensin receptor blocker; BB, β-blocker; CCB, calcium channel blocker; Aldo Antag, aldosterone antagonist. Adapted from Chobanian (2003).

thiazide diuretic drug regimen showed a significantly decreased the risk of recurrent stroke (PROGRESS Collaborative Group, 2001).

Patients should be monitored and medications adjusted monthly until the goal BP is achieved. Individuals on ACE inhibitors and ARBs should have their creatinine and potassium monitored. ACE inhibitors should only be withheld if the creatinine is greater than 30% of baseline or potassium greater than 5.6 mmol/L (Bakris, 2000). Once goal BP is reached, the patients should follow up every 3–6 months. Patients with compelling indications should be monitored more frequently.

Patients are considered to have resistant hypertension if the goal BP is not obtained with a three-drug regimen. After other identifiable causes have been excluded, consideration should be given to referral to a hypertension specialist.

REFERENCES

1. Antihypertensive and Lipid-Lowering Treatment to Prevent Heart Attack Trial (ALLHAT) Collaborative Research Group. Major outcomes in high-risk hypertensive patients randomized to angiotensin-converting enzyme inhibitor or calcium channel blocker vs diuretic: The Antihypertensive and Lipid-Lowering Treatment to Prevent Heart Attack Trial (ALLHAT). JAMA 288:2981–2997, 2002.

2. Appel LJ, Moore TJ, Obarzanek E, et al. A clinical trial of the effects of dietary patterns on blood pressure. DASH Collaborative Research Group. N Engl J Med 336:1117–1124, 1997.

3. Bakris GL, Weir MR. Angiotensin-converting enzyme inhibitor-associated elevations in serum creatinine: is this a cause for concern? Arch Intern Med 160:685–693, 2000.

4. Brenner BM, Cooper ME, de Zeeuw D, et al. Effects of losartan on renal and cardiovascular outcomes in patients with type 2 diabetes and nephropathy. N Engl J Med 345:861–869, 2001.

5. Burt VL, Whelton P, Roccella EJ, et al. Prevalence of hypertension in the US adult population. Results from the Third National Health and Nutrition Examination Survey, 1988–1991. Hypertension 25:305–313, 1995.

6. Chobanian AV, Bakris GL, Black HR, et al. The Seventh Report of the Joint National Committee on Prevention, Detection, Evaluation, and Treatment of High Blood Pressure: the JNC 7 report. JAMA 289:2560–2572, 2003.

7. CIBIS-II Investigators. The Cardiac Insufficiency Bisoprolol Study II (CIBIS-II): a randomised trial. Lancet 353:9–13, 1999.

8. Cohn JN, Tognoni G. A randomized trial of the angiotensin-receptor blocker valsartan in chronic heart failure. N Engl J Med 345:1667–1675, 2001.

9. CONSENSUS Trial Study Group. Effects of enalapril on mortality in severe congestive heart failure. Results of the Cooperative North Scandanavian

Enalapril Survival Study (CONSENSUS). N Engl J Med 316:1429–1435, 1987.

10. Dargie HJ. Effect of carvedilol on outcome after myocardial infarction in patients with left-ventricular dysfunction: the CAPRICORN randomised trial. Lancet 357:1385–1390, 2001.

11. Devereux RB, Alderman MH. Role of preclinical cardiovascular disease in the evolution from risk factor exposure to development of morbid events. Circulation 88:1444–1455, 1993.

12. Franklin SS. The concept of vascular overload in hypertension. Cardiol Clin 13:501–507, 1995.

13. GISEN (Gruppo Italiano di Studi Epidemiologici in Nefrologia Group. Randomised placebo-controlled trial of effect of ramipril on decline in glomerular filtration rate and risk of terminal renal failure in proteinuric, non-diabetic nephropathy. Lancet 349:1857–1863, 1997.

14. International Collaborative Study Group. Reduction of infarct size with the early use of timolol in acute myocardial infarction. N Engl J Med 310:9–15, 1984.

15. Izzo JL, Jr., Levy D, Black HR. Clinical Advisory Statement. Importance of systolic blood pressure in older Americans. Hypertension 35:1021–1024, 2000.

16. Jafar TH, Stark PC, Schmid CH, et al. Progression of chronic kidney disease: the role of blood pressure control, proteinuria, and angiotensin-converting enzyme inhibition: a patient-level meta-analysis. Ann Intern Med 139:244–252, 2003.

17. Lewington S, Clarke R, Qizilbash N, Peto R, Collins R. Age-specific relevance of usual blood pressure to vascular mortality: a meta-analysis of individual data for one million adults in 61 prospective studies. Lancet 360:1903–1913, 2002.

18. Madhavan S, Ooi WL, Cohen H, Alderman MH. Relation of pulse pressure and blood pressure reduction to the incidence of myocardial infarction. Hypertension 23:395–401, 1994.

19. Metoprolol CR/XL Randomised Intervention Trial in Congestive Heart Failure Investigators. Effect of metoprolol CR/XL in chronic heart failure: Metoprolol CR/XL Randomised Intervention Trial in Congestive Heart Failure (MERIT-HF). Lancet 353:2001–2007, 1999.

20. O'Rourke MF, Kelly RF. Wave reflection in the systemic circulation and its implications in ventricular function. J Hypertens 11:327–337, 1993.

21. Packer M, Bristow MR, Cohn JN, et al. The effect of carvedilol on morbidity and mortality in patients with chronic heart failure. U.S. Carvedilol Heart Failure Study Group. N Engl J Med 334:1349–1355, 1996.

22. Pfeffer MA, Braunwald E, Moye LA, et al. and , Investigators. S. Effect of captopril on mortality and morbidity in patients with left ventricular dysfunction after myocardial infarction. Results of the Survival and Ventricular Enlargement Trial. N Engl J Med 327:669–677, 1992.

23. Pitt B, Poole-Wilson PA, Segal R, et al. Effect of losartan compared with captopril on mortality in patients with symptomatic heart failure: randomised trial—the Losartan Heart Failure Survival Study ELITE II. Lancet 355:1582–1587, 2000.

24. Pitt B, Remme W, Zannad F, et al. Eplerenone, a selective aldosterone blocker, in patients with left ventricular dysfunction after myocardial infarction. N Engl J Med 348:1309–1321, 2003.

25. Pitt B, Zannad F, Remme WJ, et al. The effect of spironolactone on morbidity and mortality in patients with severe heart failure. Randomized Aldactone Evaluation Study Investigators. N Engl J Med 341:709–717, 1999.

26. PROGRESS Collaborative Group. Randomised trial of a perindopril-based blood-pressure-lowering regimen among 6,105 individuals with previous stroke or transient ischaemic attack. Lancet 358:1033–1041, 2001.

27. Ruggenenti P, Perna A, Gherardi G, et al. Renoprotective properties of ACE-inhibition in non-diabetic nephropathies with non-nephrotic proteinuria. Lancet 354:359–364, 1999.

28. Sacks FM, Svetkey LP, Vollmer WM, et al. Effects on blood pressure of reduced dietary sodium and the Dietary Approaches to Stop Hypertension (DASH) diet. DASH-Sodium Collaborative Research Group. N Engl J Med 344:3–10, 2001.

29. SHEP Cooperative Research Group. Prevention of stroke by antihypertensive drug treatment in older persons with isolated systolic hypertension. Final results of the Systolic Hypertension in the Elderly Program (SHEP). Jama 265:3255–3264, 1991.

30. SOLVD Investigators. Effect of enalapril on mortality and the development of heart failure in asymptomatic patients with reduced left ventricular ejection fractions. N Engl J Med 327:685–691, 1992.

31. SOLVD Investigators. Effect of enalapril on survival in patients with reduced left ventricular ejection fractions and congestive heart failure. N Engl J Med 325:293–302, 1991.

32. Staessen JA, Fagard R, Thijs L, et al. Randomised double-blind comparison of placebo and active treatment for older patients with isolated systolic hypertension. The Systolic Hypertension in Europe (Syst-Eur) Trial Investigators. Lancet 350:757–764, 1997.

33. Vasan RS, Beiser A, Seshadri S, et al. Residual lifetime risk for developing hypertension in middle-aged women and men: The Framingham Heart Study. Jama 287:1003–1010, 2002.

34. Wang Y, Wang QJ. The prevalence of prehypertension and hypertension among US adults according to the new joint national committee guidelines: new challenges of the old problem. Arch Intern Med 164:2126–2134, 2004.

7 Pericardial Diseases

ACUTE PERICARDITIS

Etiology and Pathophysiology

The pericardium is a fibroelastic sac that is made up of two layers (visceral and parietal), between which is contained 15 to 50 cc of fluid (Spodick, 1992). Pericarditis is a result of an inflammatory process within the pericardium. In most cases of acute pericarditis the etiology is either idiopathic or viral. Other causes include systemic autoimmune disorders, neoplastic spread, uremia, trauma, irradiation, or bacterial infection. Acute pericarditis can also occur after a myocardial infarction or following cardiac surgery. Potential sequelae of acute pericarditis include cardiac tamponade and constrictive pericarditis.

Clinical Features

Severe, retrosternal chest pain is the most common symptom of acute pericarditis. The pain is often sharp and pleuritic in nature, and may radiate to the shoulder, neck, and trapezius muscle ridges. The referred pain to the trapezius muscle ridges is the result of irritation of the phrenic nerve as it transverses the pericardium (Lange & Hillis, 2004). The intensity of the pain can vary with position, often becoming worse with recumbency and improving when the patient leans forward. Pain is also commonly exacerbated by inspiration.

The classic physical sign is a pericardial friction rub. The rub is scratchy and usually best heard along the left sternal border and during suspended respiration. There are classically three components to this rub, corresponding to the movement of the heart during atrial systole, ventricular systole, and early ventricular diastole.

The diagnosis of pericarditis is usually made by electrocardiography (ECG), with diffuse ST elevation (usually not corresponding

From: *Current Clinical Practice: Cardiology in Family Practice:*
A Practical Guide
By: S. M. Hollenberg and T. Walker © Humana Press Inc., Totowa, NJ

to an anatomic distribution, but this may not necessarily be the case in localized pericarditis) and PR segment depression. The ECG may show an evolution through four stages: stage 1—diffuse concave upsloping ST elevation and PR segment depression, stage 2—normalization of the ST and PR segments, stage 3—widespread T-wave inversions, and stage 4—normalization of the T-waves (Spodick, 1973). Stage 1 is observed in 80% of patients (Bruce & Spodick, 1980), but prompt initiation of therapy may prevent the appearance of all four stages (Spodick, 2003b). On chest radiography the cardiac silhouette may be entirely normal or may be enlarged if a pericardial effusion is present.

Elevated plasma troponin levels can be observed in acute pericarditis. Troponin release is commonly associated with male gender, ST elevations, young age, and pericardial effusion, and usually resolves within 1 week after presentation (Imazio et al., 2003). The degree of troponin elevation is roughly related to the extent of myocardial inflammatory involvement and is not a negative prognostic marker (Imazio et al., 2003).

Echocardiography can be used in patients with suspected pericarditis to evaluate for a pericardial effusion (Cheitlin et al., 2003). However, the absence of a pericardial effusion does not exclude the diagnosis of acute pericarditis.

Therapy

Treatment for acute pericarditis should be directed at the underlying cause. For patients with idiopathic pericarditis, the treatment should be directed at relieving the symptoms and decreasing the inflammation. Nonsteroidal anti-inflammatory drugs, specifically ibuprofen, are recommended as the treatment of choice for acute pericarditis (Maisch et al., 2004). The dose of ibuprofen ranges from 300 to 800 mg every 6 to 8 hours, depending on symptom severity and response to therapy. Indomethacin (50 mg three times a day) is also commonly employed. In postinfarction pericarditis, aspirin should be given at a dose of 650 mg every 4 hours for 2 to 5 days (Maisch et al., 2004). Colchicine can also be used, either as monotherapy or in combination with nonsteroidal agents (Maisch et al., 2004). Steroids are recommended only for refractory disease, connective tissue disease, or uremic pericarditis (Maisch et al., 2004). To ensure resolution, patients should be followed up on an outpatient basis. A subsequent echocardiogram is recommended if an effusion recurs or if pericardial constriction is suspected (Maisch et al., 2004).

Pericardiocentesis is indicated for tamponade, a high suspicion of purulent or neoplastic pericarditis, or for large or symptomatic effusions that persist despite medical therapy for more than 1 week (Maisch et al., 2004).

CARDIAC TAMPONADE
Etiology and Pathophysiology

Cardiac tamponade is a life-threatening emergency that results from an accumulation of fluid within the pericardium that compresses all the chambers of the heart. The causes of tamponade are the same as pericardial effusions, which include pericarditis, malignancy, trauma, dissecting aortic aneurysm, tuberculosis, systemic lupus erythematosus, uremia, and following surgical or diagnostic procedures.

The pericardium normally has some elasticity, but there is a limit after which pericardial pressure rises quickly. The consequences of pericardial fluid depend on the rate of accumulation, pericardial compliance, and patient blood volume. As little as 200 mL to as much as 2 L can cause tamponade (Reddy et al., 1978). Once the pericardium becomes inelastic, the heart and pericardial contents must compete for a fixed intrapericardial volume (Santamore et al., 1990; Spodick, 1998).

As fluid continues to accumulate, compensatory mechanisms include increased right-sided pressures to maintain cardiac filling, tachycardia, increased ejection fraction, and increased peripheral vascular tone, all of which are mediated by increased sympathetic tone. With increased compression of the heart chambers, the gradient for cardiac inflow is reduced. The right ventricle and atrium are affected by the compressive effect during times of lowest pressure (atrial relaxation and ventricular diastole). As the intrapericardial pressure increases, the heart is compressed throughout the cardiac cycle. With inspiration, there is an increase in venous return and volume in the right ventricle, which causes the interventricular septum to bulge into the left ventricle, thus decreasing stroke volume and cardiac output (Spodick, 2003a). With further decompensation, blood pressure is decreased, and shock can occur.

Clinical Features

The symptoms of cardiac tamponade result from decreased cardiac output and pulmonary congestion. Symptoms can be dramatic, but are often nonspecific, and include dyspnea, chest pain, weakness, orthopnea, cough, and dysphagia.

The classic physical examination findings are jugular venous distension, hypotension and muffled heart sounds, known as Beck's triad. The jugular venous pulsations show a prominent **x** (systolic) descent, and a markedly decreased or absent **y** (diastolic) descent, reflecting impaired diastolic filling. Other findings include tachycardia, tachypnea, and pulsus paradoxus. Pulsus paradoxus is defined as a decrease in systolic blood pressure greater than 10 mmHg with inspiration, and results from increased right-sided filling with inspiration at the expense of left-sided filling, decreasing stroke volume. Pulsus paradoxus can also be seen in chronic obstructive pulmonary diseases, pulmonary embolism, and hypovolemia. Hypotension is a late sign.

Findings on ECG associated with cardiac tamponade include low voltage and electrical alternans, changing electrical axis, which results from swinging of the heart within the pericardial fluid, although the ECG may be unremarkable except for tachycardia. The chest x-ray may show an enlarged cardiac silhouette ("water bottle" heart).

Echocardiography is indicated in all patients with suspected tamponade, not only to document the presence of a pericardial effusion but to define its hemodynamic significance. Significant changes in transvalvular flow velocities with respiration (>25%) are the echocardiographic equivalent of a paradoxical pulse, and indicate that an effusion is hemodynamically significant. Inferior vena cava plethora is indicative of high venous pressures, and is the most sensitive finding on echocardiography (Himelman et al., 1988). With tamponade, loss of the transmural pressure gradient in the right atrium and right ventricle can lead to diastolic collapse. Right ventricular collapse is more specific for tamponade than right atrial collapse (Kronzon et al., 1983a,b).

Cardiac tamponade is a hemodynamic diagnosis. The diagnosis is made definitively by demonstration of elevation and equalization of right atrial mean, right ventricle diastolic, pulmonary artery diastolic, and pulmonary artery wedge pressure (within 5 mm of one another), which entails right heart catheterization.

Therapy

Fluid therapy and vasopressor support are temporizing measures in patients with cardiac tamponade; definitive therapy requires removal of pericardial fluid. The heart is maximally stimulated by sympathetic drive, and exogenous inotropic agents add little (Spodick, 2003a).

Patients with tamponade physiology should be considered for emergent pericardiocentesis. Because of the steepness of the pericardial compliance curve, prompt relief can be obtained with removal of only a small amount of fluid. Pericardiocentesis is usually not effective applicable in penetrating wounds, ruptured ventricular aneurysms, or dissecting aortas (Cheitlin et al., 2003). For patients requiring prolonged drainage, a multihole pigtail drainage catheter can be left in place until drainage is decreased to less than 50 cc per day (Spodick, 2003a). The fluid can also be removed by surgical creation of a pericardial window. This is preferred when biopsies are required, the fluid is loculated, the fluid has re-accumulated, or the patient is coagulopathic.

CONSTRICTIVE PERICARDITIS
Etiology and Pathophysiology

Constrictive pericarditis results from an inflammatory process that calcifies and thickens the pericardium. The scarring and inelasticity interferes with diastolic filling and ultimately decreases cardiac output. Constrictive pericarditis can occur after any pericardial disease. Most cases are idiopathic, and probably result from chronic pericarditis. Tuberculosis is a much less common cause in the United States than worldwide. Other etiologies include radiation, postsurgical, malignancy, uremia, posttraumatic, and connective tissue disorders.

The rigid, noncompliant pericardium in constrictive pericarditis restricts ventricular filling. Initially, there is early rapid unrestricted diastolic filling. Filling ceases at the end of the first third of diastole when the intracardiac volume reaches its limit as a result of the rigid pericardium. The end-diastolic pressure and the atrial pressure are elevated and nearly equal, whereas the end-diastolic volumes are reduced. Stroke volume and cardiac output decrease, resulting in both left and right heart failure.

Characteristic hemodynamic findings include a dip and plateau "square root" sign on the right ventricular pressure tracing and the M or W configuration. The square root sign reflects the early rapid diastolic filling with sudden cessation as the pericardium reaches its compliance limit. On the venous pressure tracing, the **a** and **v** waves are prominent and the **x** and **y** descents are steep, producing an M or W configuration. The cardiac volume is fixed by the stiff pericardium and therefore the intrathoracic changes with respiration are not transmitted to the heart, although the pulmonary vein and systemic veins are affected. With inspiration, the filling-pressure gradient from the pulmonary veins to the left ventricle is decreased, resulting in decreased mitral flow velocities. With less filling of the left ventricle, the interventricular septum shifts to the left, allowing redistribution of the blood into the right ventricle. This is reflected in increased tricuspid inflow and diastolic hepatic vein flow velocities. The opposite occurs with expiration.

Pericardial constriction presents insidiously. Dyspnea on exertion, decreased exercise tolerance and fatigue are usually the first symptoms. Other symptoms may include nonspecific abdominal symptoms and weight loss. As the constriction progresses, dyspnea worsens.

Physical findings include ascites, pulsatile hepatomegaly, and elevated jugular venous pressure. The systolic **x** descent is steep owing to increased venous pressures, and the early diastolic descent is steep as well because of rapid early diastolic filling. Kussmaul's sign, a paradoxical rise in jugular venous pressure during inspiration, was historically described in constrictive pericarditis, but occurs in only a minority of patients. The characteristic auscultatory finding is a mid-diastolic pericardial knock, which represents a sudden cessation in ventricular inflow.

There are no specific findings on ECG for constrictive pericarditis, but low voltage, and T-wave inversion or flattening may be seen. Chest radiograph may show pericardial calcifications, biatrial enlargement, and pleural effusions.

Echocardiography with Doppler should be performed on all patients suspected of having constrictive pericarditis (Cheitlin et al., 2003). Echocardiographic features of constrictive pericarditis may include a thickened pericardium and a septal bounce caused by rapid cessation of ventricular filling. The inferior vena cava and hepatic vein may be dilated. Doppler is used to assess diastolic filling. In constrictive pericarditis, the rapid early diastolic filling is reflected in the high early inflow velocities, with very little contribution from atrial contraction. Doppler may also show respiratory variations in transmitral, transtricuspid, pulmonary, and hepatic flows.

Cardiac catheterization is performed if echocardiography is nondiagnostic. The prominent **x** and **y** descent, dip, and plateau in right ventricular diastolic pressure (square root sign), and impaired diastolic filling are seen with right heart catheterization. Catheterization can also show the equalization of the end-diastolic pressures of the heart. Computed tomography and magnetic resonance imaging are both noninvasive and sensitive methods for confirming pericardial thickening once the characteristic physiology has been demonstrated. Diagnosing constrictive pericarditis (Masui et al., 1992; Wang et al., 2003).

Therapy

For most patients, pericardial stripping is recommended for constrictive pericarditis. Patients with mild constriction or advanced disease may not benefit from pericardiectomy. Predictors of adverse outcomes following pericardiectomy include advanced age, renal dysfunction, left ventricular dysfunction, pulmonary hypertension, hyponatremia, and disease owing to radiation therapy (Bertog et al., 2004; Ling et al., 1999).

REFERENCES

1. Bertog SC, Thambidorai SK, Parakh K, et al. Constrictive pericarditis: etiology and cause-specific survival after pericardiectomy. J Am Coll Cardiol 43: 1445–1452, 2004.
2. Bruce MA, Spodick DH. Atypical electrocardiogram in acute pericarditis: characteristics and prevalence. J Electrocardiol 13:61–66, 1980.
3. Cheitlin MD, Armstrong WF, Aurigemma GP, et al. ACC/AHA/ASE 2003 guideline update for the clinical application of echocardiography: summary article: a report of the American College of Cardiology/American Heart Association Task Force on Practice Guidelines (ACC/AHA/ASE Committee to Update the 1997 Guidelines for the Clinical Application of Echocardiography). Circulation 108: 1146–1162, 2003.

4. Himelman RB, Kircher B, Rockey DC, Schiller NB. Inferior vena cava plethora with blunted respiratory response: a sensitive echocardiographic sign of cardiac tamponade. J Am Coll Cardiol 12: 1470–1477, 1988.

5. Imazio M, Demichelis B, Cecchi E, Belli R, Ghisio A, Bobbio M, Trinchero R. Cardiac troponin I in acute pericarditis. J Am Coll Cardiol 42: 2144–2148, 2003.

6. Kronzon I, Cohen ML, Winer HE. Contribution of echocardiography to the understanding of the pathophysiology of cardiac tamponade. J Am Coll Cardiol 1: 1180–1182, 1983a.

7. Kronzon I, Cohen ML, Winer HE. Diastolic atrial compression: a sensitive echocardiographic sign of cardiac tamponade. J Am Coll Cardiol 2: 770–775, 1983b.

8. Lange RA, Hillis LD. Clinical practice. Acute pericarditis. N Engl J Med 351:2195–2202, 2004.

9. Ling LH, Oh JK, Schaff HV, et al. Constrictive pericarditis in the modern era: evolving clinical spectrum and impact on outcome after pericardiectomy. Circulation 100: 1380–1386, 1999.

10. Maisch B, Seferovic PM, Ristic AD, et al. Guidelines on the diagnosis and management of pericardial diseases executive summary; The Task force on the diagnosis and management of pericardial diseases of the European society of cardiology. Eur Heart J 25:587–610, 2004.

11. Masui T, Finck S, Higgins CB. Constrictive pericarditis and restrictive cardiomyopathy: evaluation with MR imaging. Radiology 182:369–373, 1992.

12. Reddy PS, Curtiss EI, O'Toole JD, Shaver JA. Cardiac tamponade: hemodynamic observations in man. Circulation 58:265–272, 1978.

13. Santamore WP, Li KS, Nakamoto T, Johnston WE. Effects of increased pericardial pressure on the coupling between the ventricles. Cardiovasc Res 24: 768–776, 1990.

14. Spodick DH. Acute cardiac tamponade. N Engl J Med 349: 684–690, 2003a.

15. Spodick DH. Acute pericarditis: current concepts and practice. JAMA 289:1150–1153, 2003b.

16. Spodick DH. Diagnostic electrocardiographic sequences in acute pericarditis. Significance of PR segment and PR vector changes. Circulation 48:575–580, 1973.

17. Spodick DH. Macrophysiology, microphysiology, and anatomy of the pericardium: a synopsis. Am Heart J 124: 1046–1051, 1992.

18. Spodick DH. Pathophysiology of cardiac tamponade. Chest 113: 1372–1378, 1998.

19. Wang ZJ, Reddy GP, Gotway MB, Yeh BM, Hetts SW, Higgins CB. CT and MR imaging of pericardial disease. Radiographics 23: S167–-180, 2003.

8   Stable Angina

DEFINITION

Myocardial ischemia results from an imbalance of oxygen supply and oxygen demand. Classically, myocardial ischemia has been divided into categories including stable angina, unstable angina, and myocardial infarction (MI). Typical angina is exertional, and is relieved promptly by rest or nitroglycerin. Stable angina occurs reproducibly with a similar level of exertion, in a pattern that is unchanged over the previous 6 months. Unstable angina consists of ischemic symptoms that are more frequent, severe, or prolonged than the patient's usual angina, are more difficult to control with drugs, or are occurring at rest or minimal exertion. Cardiac biomarkers are not elevated. When cardiac biomarkers are elevated and there is evidence of myocardial damage, the term *infarction* is used.

PATHOPHYSIOLOGY

The heart is an aerobic organ with only a limited capacity for anaerobic glycolysis. It makes use of oxygen avidly and efficiently, extracting 70 to 80% of the oxygen from coronary arterial blood (Braunwald, 1971). Because the heart extracts oxygen nearly maximally independent of demand, increases in demand must be met by commensurate increases in coronary blood flow. The myocardial requirement for oxygen, and hence for oxygenated blood, is affected by three major variables: heart rate, myocardial wall stress, and contractility. Myocardial wall stress is a function of the radius, and the intraventricular pressure, which is highly dependent on ventricular afterload (*see* Fig. 1).

Coronary blood flow depends on coronary perfusion pressure (CPP) and filling time. Because coronary perfusion occurs primarily

From: *Current Clinical Practice: Cardiology in Family Practice:*
A Practical Guide
By: S. M. Hollenberg and T. Walker © Humana Press Inc., Totowa, NJ

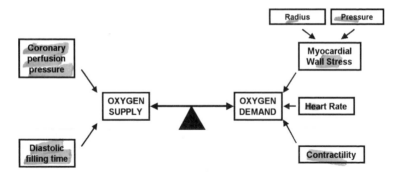

Fig. 1. Determinants of myocardial oxygen supply and demand.

in diastole, the relevant pressure gradient is aortic diastolic pressure minus left ventricular (LV) diastolic pressure. Filling time is directly related to heart rate.

Myocardial ischemia usually develops in the setting of obstructive atherosclerotic coronary artery disease, which limits blood supply. The pathophysiology of unstable coronary syndromes and MI usually involves dynamic partial or complete occlusion of an epicardial coronary artery because of acute intracoronary thrombus formation (DeWood, 1986).

A number of factors can increase myocardial oxygen demand, including tachycardia, hypertension, and increased catecholamines resulting from stress. Similarly, many factors could contribute to limitation of oxygen supply, particularly in the setting of hemodynamic instability. These factors include hypotension, decreasing CPP, and tachycardia, limiting diastolic filling time. In addition, anemia and hypoxemia can limit the amount of oxygen delivered to the heart. Coronary vasospasm may also play a role in some patients. Elevation of LV pressures by heart failure can both increase demand and reduce CPP.

DIAGNOSIS

Signs And Symptoms

Myocardial ischemia is most commonly manifested as constant substernal chest tightness or pressure. The pain is typically left-sided and may radiate to the throat and jaw or to the left shoulder and

Table 1
Canadian Cardiovascular Society Classification of Angina

Class	I	Symptoms only with strenuous activity
Class	II	Slight limitation in ordinary physical activity
Class	III	Marked limitation in ordinary physical activity
Class	IV	Symptoms with any activity or at rest

left arm and is often accompanied by acute onset of dyspnea and diaphoresis. Angina may occasionally be right-sided, interscapular, or perceived in the epigastrium. The severity of anginal symptoms can be rated from class I to IV using the Canadian Cardiovascular society classification (*see* Table 1).

Because other syndromes may mimic angina, it is important to consider them in the differential diagnosis. These include dissecting aortic aneurysm; pericarditis; pleuritis; pulmonary processes such as pulmonary embolism, pneumonia, and pneumothorax; gastrointestinal (GI) processes such as esophageal or peptic ulcer disease and cholecystitis; musculoskeletal pain; and costochondritis. Other heart diseases (valvular heart disease, cardiomyopathies, myocarditis) not attributable to coronary artery stenosis may also cause substernal chest tightness and should also be included in the differential diagnosis.

The physical examination, although sometimes insensitive and nonspecific, especially in the patient with multisystem illness or with pre-existing LV dysfunction, may be helpful in confirming the diagnosis. Elevated jugular veins signal right ventricular diastolic pressure elevation, and the appearance of pulmonary crackles (in the absence of pulmonary disease) indicates elevated LV filling pressures secondary to depressed LV function. A systolic bulge occasionally can be palpated on the precordium in the area of the apex of the heart, representing contact of an ischemic dyskinetic segment of the left ventricle with the chest wall. During the ischemic episode, auscultation of the precordium may reveal the presence of a fourth heart sound, indicative of a noncompliant left ventricle. With extensive myocardial dysfunction, a third heart sound may be present. A murmur of mitral regurgitation attributable to papillary muscle dysfunction may also emerge.

The Electrocardiogram

The electrocardiographic (ECG) abnormalities in myocardial ischemia vary widely and depend in large part on the extent and nature of coronary stenosis and the presence of collateral blood flow to ischemic zones. A full consideration of ECG interpretation is beyond the scope of this chapter. ECG findings of ischemia depend on its duration, extent and localization, as well as the presence of other underlying abnormalities.

The most prominent ECG changes with ischemia occur in the ST segment, which is normally isoelectric because the cells have the same membrane potential during repolarization. Cellular ischemia lowers the resting potential and thus creates a voltage gradient between normal and ischemic areas, which shifts the ST segment. In transmural ischemia, the ST segment is shifted toward the epicardial layers, producing ST elevation (also known as "injury current.") With subendocardial ischemia, the ST segment is shifted toward the endocardium layers, producing ST depression. Classic angina produces ST depression.

The pattern of ECG changes may give a guide to the area and extent of infarction. The number of leads involved broadly reflects the extent of myocardium involved. Although localization of the area of ischemia is more accurate when the ST segments are elevated than when they are depressed, the general pattern is similar. Anterior ischemia is manifest in leads V_1–V_4, inferior ischemia in leads II,III, and aVF, and lateral ischemia in leads I, aVL, V_5, and V_6.

The ECG diagnosis of ischemia can be difficult in the presence of conduction abnormalities, most prominently left bundle branch block. ST depression can also be caused by medications, digitalis in particular, electrolyte disorders, most prominently hypokalemia. LV hypertrophy may also result in ST depression—the so-called "strain" pattern. Cardiomyopathy, myocarditis, and cerebrovascular events can also cause ST depression, as can supraventricular tachycardias, even in the absence of coronary artery disease (CAD).

Differential Diagnosis

The differential diagnosis of chest discomfort is broad and includes GI, pulmonary, musculoskeletal, and neurological causes, which can sometimes be difficult to distinguish from cardiac symptoms because the heart shares some sensory innervation with other thoracic organs.

Pericarditis can present like ischemia, although the pain of pericarditis is more commonly sharp and pleuritic, and may be positional. Prominent GI causes of chest pain include esophageal disorders such as reflux, spasm, other motility disorders, and esophageal rupture, peptic ulcer disease, cholecystitis, and pancreatitis (Voskuil, 1996). Pulmonary causes include pneumonia, pulmonary embolism, pleuritis, pneumothorax, and pulmonary hypertension. Musculoskeletal causes such as costochondritis and other chest wall symptoms merit consideration. Thoracic disk herniation and zoster can also present with chest discomfort.

Stress Testing

Patients with an intermediate probability of obstructive CAD should be considered for stress testing to establish the diagnosis. Exercise treadmill testing is preferred, unless they are unable to exercise or the resting ECG is abnormal, in which case alternative techniques may be considered. Myocardial perfusion imaging or echocardiography can be added to improve sensitivity or specificity, and is especially useful with resting ECG abnormalities. Imaging also allows for better localization of ischemic areas.

Pharmacological testing using adenosine or dipyridamole with myocardial perfusion imaging can identify relative perfusion defects suggestive of significant coronary stenosis. Dipyridamole and adenosine dilate the coronary microvasculature and markedly increase blood flow. The flow increases less through stenotic arteries, creating heterogeneous myocardial perfusion, which can be detected using the perfusion tracer. Although this mechanism can (and often does) produce reversible perfusion defects independent of myocardial ischemia, in some patients, true myocardial ischemia can occur because of coronary steal.

TREATMENT

As previously noted, myocardial ischemia results from an imbalance of myocardial oxygen supply and demand. Patients with a history of stable angina who develop chest pain may be treated by removal of provocative stimuli that can increase myocardial oxygen consumption or lead to compromised coronary blood flow, if these factors can be identified. For example, correction of hypoxia, anemia, hypovolemia, tachycardia, or labile hypertension may be sufficient to control anginal episodes. Often overlooked are fever, infection, anxiety, stress, activity, and the work of breathing.

Treatment of stable angina entails a combination of therapeutic interventions aimed at relieving symptoms and lifestyle interventions to minimize the potential complications. The mnemonic ABCDE mixes the two, serving to emphasize the point that acute interventions are only the prelude to secondary prevention (chronic angina guidelines). This mnemonic goes as follows:

- Aspirin
- Anti-anginals
- ACE inhibitors
- β-Blockers
- Blood pressure control
- Cholesterol reduction
- Cigarettes: smoking cessation program
- Calcium channel blockers
- Dietary modification
- Diabetes management
- Education
- Exercise

Aspirin

Aspirin is the best-known and the most widely used of all the antiplatelet agents because of low cost and relatively low toxicity. Use of salicylates to treat CAD in the United States was first reported in 1953 (Craven, 1953) Aspirin inhibits the production of thromboxane A_2 by irreversibly acetylating the serine residue of the enzyme prostaglandin H_2 synthetase.

Reduction of death or nonfatal MI in patients with unstable angina and non-ST elevation MI has been well established in several large randomized clinical trials (Lewis, 1983; Theroux, 1988). In addition to its use in acute clinical settings, aspirin has also been shown to be beneficial in preventing cardiovascular events when administered as secondary prevention in patients after acute MI and as primary prevention in subjects with no prior history of vascular disease

(Steering Committee of the Physicians' Health Study Research Group, 1989).

The most widely used and effective dose of aspirin in cardiovascular disease (CVD) is between 81 mg and 325 mg daily. Despite the fact aspirin blocks thromboxane preferentially to prostacyclin at low doses and thus has a more profound antiplatelet effect, high-dose aspirin has been found to be as effective as low-dose aspirin in prevention of cardiovascular death, MI, and stroke (Platelet Receptor Inhibition in Ischemic Syndrome Management in Patients Limited by Unstable Signs and Symptoms (PRISM-PLUS) Study Investigators, 1998), which may suggest that besides its antiplatelet effects, the anti-inflammatory effects of aspirin play a role as well (Ridker, 1997). Once begun, aspirin should probably be continued indefinitely. Toxicity with aspirin is mostly GI; enteric-coated preparations may minimize these side effects.

Anti-Anginals: Nitrates

Nitroglycerin is a mainstay of therapy for angina because of its efficacy and rapid onset of action. The most important anti-anginal effect of nitroglycerin is preferential dilation of venous capacitance vessels, decreasing venous return. A reduction in myocardial oxygen demand and consumption results from the reduction of LV volume and arterial pressure primarily due to reduced preload (Cohn, 1974). At higher doses, in some patients, nitroglycerin relaxes arterial smooth muscle as well, causing a modest decrease in afterload, which also contributes to wall stress (Cohn, 1974). In addition, nitroglycerin can epicardial coronary arteries, and nitroglycerin redistributes coronary blood flow to ischemic regions by dilating collateral vessels. Nitroglycerin has antithrombotic and antiplatelet effects as well.

The quickest route of administration of nitroglycerin is sublingual. Sublingual doses of 0.4 mg may be administered every 5 to 10 minutes for a total of three doses, if required to control pain. Topical or oral nitrates may be used for chronic therapy.

Because of its hemodynamic actions, systemic blood pressure (BP) may fall after nitroglycerin administration, so frequent BP checks are required. Hypotension, should it occur, can normally be resolved by placing the patient in the Trendelenburg position and by giving intravenous saline boluses.

Angiotensin-Converting Enzyme Inhibitors

Angiotensin-converting enzyme (ACE) generates angiotensin II from angiotensin I and also catalyzes the breakdown of bradykinin. Thus, ACE inhibitors can decrease circulating angiotensin II levels and increase levels of bradykinin, which in turn stimulates production of nitric oxide by endothelial nitric oxide synthase. In the vasculature, ACE inhibition promotes vasodilation, and tends to inhibit smooth muscle proliferation, platelet aggregation, and thrombosis.

The major hemodynamic effect of ACE inhibition is afterload reduction, which is most important as an influence of myocardial oxygen demand in patients with impaired LV function. The Heart Outcomes Prevention Evaluation (HOPE) trial randomized 9297 patients with documented vascular disease or those at high risk for atherosclerosis (diabetes plus at least one other risk factor) in the absence of heart failure to treatment with the tissue-selective ACE inhibitor ramipril (target dose 10 mg/day) or placebo (Yusuf, 2000). and showed a 22% reduction in the combined endpoint of cardiovascular death, MI, and stroke (Yusuf, 2000). Cardiovascular risk reduction in patients with stable angina was also found using perindopril in the EUROPA trial (Fox, 2003). Recently, however, the Prevention of Events With Angiotensin-Converting Enzyme Inhibition (PEACE) trial compared trandolapril with placebo in 8290 patients with stable CAD, and found no significant difference in death, MI, or need for revascularization (Braunwald, 2004). The reason for these differences remains unclear; lipid control was better in the PEACE trial, but differences in the drugs cannot be excluded. Interestingly, in all of the trials, ACE inhibition reduced the onset of new diabetes; the mechanism for this effect remains uncertain.

On the basis of these data, the latest American College of Cardiology/American Heart Association guidelines recommend use of ACE inhibitors in patients with stable angina and LV dysfunction or diabetics without severe renal disease, with consideration for routine secondary prevention for patients with known CAD (Gibbons, 2003).

β-Blockers

The rationale for administration of β-blockers during ischemic episodes derives from their negative chronotropic and negative inotropic properties. Heart rate and contractility are two of the three major determinants of myocardial oxygen consumption. By altering these variables, myocardial ischemia can be attenuated significantly (Frishman, 1983). These agents are particularly effective in patients with angina who remain tachycardic or hypertensive (or both) and in patients with supraventricular tachycardia complicating myocardial ischemia. Rapid control can be achieved by intravenous administration of metoprolol, a β_1-selective blocker, in 5 mg increments every 5 minutes up to 15 mg. Thereafter, 25 to 50 mg every 6 hours can be given orally. β-Blockers should be used with caution in patients with marginal blood pressure, pre-existing bradycardia, arterioventricular nodal conduction disturbances, and evidence for LV failure, as well as those with bronchospastic disease. Diabetes is not a contraindication to β-blocker therapy, and in fact the absolute risk reduction may be greater in these patients since they are at higher cardiovascular risk.

Blood Pressure Control

Antihypertensive therapy has been shown to reduce the incidence of MI by 20 to 25%, of heart failure by 50% or more, and of stroke by 35 to 40% (Neal, 2000). Thus, BP control is of obvious importance in both the acute and chronic management of angina. A full consideration of BP control can be found elsewhere in this volume. In patients with coronary artery disease, the goal BP is less than 130/80 mmHg (Chobanian, 2003).

Cholesterol Reduction

There is extensive epidemiological, laboratory, and clinical evidence linking cholesterol and CAD. Total cholesterol level has been linked to the development of CAD events with a continuous and graded relation (Lipid Research Clinics Program, 1984). Most of this risk is the result of low-density lipoprotein (LDL) cholesterol. A number of large primary and secondary prevention trials have shown that LDL cholesterol lowering is associated with a reduced risk of coronary disease events. Earlier lipid-lowering trials used bile-acid sequestrants (cholestyramine), fibric-acid derivatives (gemfibrozil and clofibrate), or niacin in addition to diet. The reduction in total cholesterol in these early trials was 6 to 15% and was accompanied by a consistent trend toward a reduction in fatal and nonfatal coronary events (Frick, 1987).

More impressive results have been achieved using hydroxy-methylglutaryl coenzyme A reductase inhibitors (statins). Statins have been demonstrated to decrease the rate of adverse ischemic events in patients with documented CAD in the 4S trial (Scandinavian Simvastatin Survival Study Group, 1994). as well as in the CARE study (Sacks, 1996) and the LIPID trial (Long-Term Intervention with Pravastatin in in Ischaemic Disease [LIPID] study group, 1998). On the basis of these trials, the last National Cholesterol Education Program guidelines proposed an LDL cholesterol level less than 130 mg/dL as a treatment goal (Gibbons, 2003), but an update based on more recent data recommended an even lower LDL target of less than 100 mg/dL (Grundy, 2004). Maximum benefit may require management of other lipid abnormalities (elevated triglycerides, low HDL cholesterol) and treatment of other atherogenic risk factors.

Since the publication of those guidelines, however, results of several new trials have emerged. The PROVE-IT trial randomized 4162 patients with acute coronary syndromes to pravastatin (40 mg daily, standard therapy) 80 mg of atorvastatin daily (80 mg, intensive therapy). LDL cholesterol was 125 mg/dL at baseline, and was lowered more in the intensive therapy group (to 62 mg/dL) than in the standard therapy group (95 mg/dl). This reduction was associated with a significant reduction in primary endpoint (a composite of death, MI, unstable angina, revascularization, and stroke), from 26.3 to 22.4%, $p = 0.005$ (Cannon, 2004). Another trial, the REVERSAL trial, showed that intensive lipid-lowering treatment with atorvastatin, which lowered LDL cholesterol from 150 mg/dL to 79 mg/dL reduced progression of coronary atherosclerosis, as assessed by intracoronary ultrasound, compared with a moderate regimen that lowered LDL to 110 mg/dL (Nissen, 2004). These trials suggest that such patients benefit from early and continued lowering of LDL cholesterol to levels substantially below current target levels.

Cigarettes: Smoking Cessation Program

Cigarette smoking is the most important alterable risk factor contributing to premature morbidity and mortality in the United States. As many as 30% of all CAD deaths in the United States each year are attributable to cigarette smoking, and smoking also doubles the risk of ischemic stroke. Smoking acts synergistically with other risk factors, and the risk is strongly dose-related.

Smoking cessation decreases the risk of coronary morbidity and mortality as well as stroke, with a diminution of risk that starts very soon after quitting, but also progresses over time. Benefits can, however, be obtained from smoking cessation even after many years of smoking and after presentation of smoking related disease. In fact, development of clinical illness often represents a "teachable moment" during which patients are highly motivated to change their lifestyle. The provision of a multicomponent smoking cessation program, with or without pharmacotherapy, is associated with a 50% long-term (>1 year) smoking cessation rate in patients who have been hospitalized with a coronary event, and telephone-based counseling has the potential to increase this to 70% (Ockene, 1997).

There is overwhelming evidence demonstrating both the cardio-vascular hazards of smoking and the prompt benefit that occurs with smoking cessation. The provision of advice alone significantly increases the smoking cessation rate, and even minimal counseling yields a further benefit. Intervention with patients who have already suffered a cardiac event yields particularly striking benefits. The smoking status of all patients should be assessed and appropriate intervention offered to those who smoke.

Calcium Channel Blockers

Non-dihydropyridine calcium channel blockers (CCBs; verapamil and diltiazem) also have negative chronotropic and inotropic effects, and can be used to control myocardial oxygen demand in patients with ischemia. Both can be given as intravenous boluses, starting with low doses (diltiazem 10–20 mg, verapamil 2.5 mg), and can then be infused continuously.

CCBs are particularly useful in the setting of coronary vasospasm, because they cause direct dilation of coronary vascular smooth muscle. Vasospasm can produce variant angina in patients with mild or no CAD (Prinzmetal's angina), or aggravate ischemia in patients with atherosclerotic coronary stenoses that are subcritical but serve as sites of vasospasm, possibly as a consequence of abnormalities of the underlying smooth muscle or derangements in endothelial physiology (Oliva, 1973). The illicit use of cocaine is increasingly being recognized as a cause of coronary vasospasm leading to angina and myocardial ischemia. Coronary vasospasm usually presents with ST elevation associated with chest pain, and can be difficult to differentiate from vessel closure because of coronary thrombosis. Consideration of the clinical setting, rapid fluctuation of ST segments, and prompt resolution with nitrates can provide useful clues. Variant angina attributable to vasospasm responds well to treatment with CCBs.

Short-acting dihydropyridine calcium blockers, however, have been associated with increased cardiovascular risk with long-term use, and should in general be avoided. A similar risk has not been shown, however, for extended release preparations (Stason, 1999).

Dietary Modification

Dietary management is of clear importance for the management of heart disease. On a population level, limitation of dietary saturated fat to less than 10% of energy and cholesterol to less than 300 mg per day, but specific recommendations for individuals should be based on cholesterol and lipoprotein levels and the presence of diabetes and other risk factors. Studies support a major benefit on BP of consuming vegetables, fruits, and low-fat dairy products, as well as limiting salt intake (<6 g/day) and alcohol (no more than two drinks per day for men and one for women) and maintaining a healthy body weight. Consumption of at least two fish servings per week is now recommended on the basis of evidence that consumption of omega-3 fatty acids confers cardiovascular benefits (Krauss, 2000).

Obesity is being increasingly recognized as an important risk factor for CAD and thus an important target for preventive strategies. Being overweight is associated with an increased incidence and prevalence of hypertension and diabetes before and during adulthood as well as with the later development of CVD in adults. A constellation of risk factors known as the metabolic syndrome (abdominal obesity, high triglycerides and low HDL, hypertension, and insulin resistance) confers a particularly high risk of cardiac disease and complications. When body mass index (BMI) is excessive, caloric intake should be less than energy expended in physical activity to reduce BMI. In general, relative caloric restriction sufficient to produce weight reductions between 5 and 10% can reduce the risk factors for CVD and stroke. Weight-loss programs that result in a slow but steady weight reduction (1 to 2 lb per week for up to 6 months) appear to be at least as efficacious as diets with more rapid initial weight loss over the long term and may be more effective in promoting the behavioral changes needed to maintain weight loss (Krauss, 2000).

Diabetes Management

The prevalence of diabetes in the United States is increasing rapidly, as is the incidence of abnormal glucose tolerance, likely driven by the increasing frequency of obesity and sedentary lifestyles. Both individuals with impaired glucose tolerance and those with frank diabetes are at high risk for CVD. Patients with diabetes are at increased risk of CVD and also have an increased risk of cardiac events once the diagnosis of CAD has been established. The prevalence of, incidence of, and mortality from all forms of CVD are two- to eightfold higher in persons with diabetes than in those without diabetes (Gibbons, 2003). In fact, the projected cardiovascular mortality of a diabetic without known CAD is equivalent to that of a nondiabetic patient who has experienced an MI, thus leading to the designation of diabetes as a "coronary risk equivalent." Additional cardiac risk factors amplify the risk in patients with diabetes.

This increased risk impacts both preventive and therapeutic strategies for patients with diabetes and angina. Treatment of other cardiac risk factors, especially hypertension and hyperlipidemia, should be vigorous. Target LDL cholesterol should be less than 100 mg/dL and maybe lower than that. Intensive drug therapy is clearly protective in diabetic patients, and thus all people with diabete should therefore have their BP lowered to below 130/80 mmHg (Chobanian, 2003).

Tight glycemic control is important as well. In patients with type 1 diabetes, the prospective Diabetes Control and Complications Trial showed that strict glycemic control with intensive insulin therapy can both delay the onset of microvascular complications and slow progression of complications already present (Diabetes Control and Complications Trial Research Group, 1993). Cardiovascular events were decreased from 5.4 to 3.2%, but this did not reach statistical significance (Diabetes Control and Complications Trial Research Group, 1993). In type II diabetics, the United Kingdom Prospective Diabetes Study (UKPDS) also showed a reduced risk of microvascular disease with strict glycemic control (UKPDS Group, 1998).

Education

Education is of clear importance to optimize the efficacy of therapeutic and preventive measures. This is as true for physicians and other health workers as it is for the patients themselves. In addition to published literature and patient education materials, a number of web sites, including those of the American College of Cardiology (www.acc.org), the American Heart Association (www.american heart.org), and the National Institute of Heart, Lung, and Blood (www.nhlbi.nih.gov) provide useful resources.

Exercise

Regular physical activity prevents the development of CAD (CAD) and reduces symptoms in patients with established CVD. Moderate to intense aerobic activity, with achievement of 80–85% of maximum predicted heart rate, provides optimal cardiac benefits, but lesser activity is also protective. Physical activity reduces insulin resistance and glucose intolerance, and is an important adjunct to diet for achieving and maintaining weight loss.

Comprehensive, exercise-based cardiac rehabilitation reduces mortality rates in patients after MI, although the rate of recurrent infarction is not significantly altered. Regular exercise in patients with stable CAD has been shown to improve myocardial perfusion and to retard disease progression (Thompson, 2003). In fact, a recent randomized trial of patients with angiographic coronary disease showed that compared with percutaneous intervention, a 12-month program of regular physical exercise in selected patients with stable CAD resulted in superior event-free survival and exercise capacity (Hambrecht, 2004).

REVASCULARIZATION

If anginal symptoms persist despite maximal medical therapy, coronary angiography with an aim toward possible revascularization should be considered. One must keep in mind that coronary angiography is not a therapeutic intervention, but a diagnostic test. Angiography is of little tangible value if there are no viable revascularization options.

Revascularization can be performed by coronary artery bypass grafting (CABG), in which autologous arteries or veins are used to reroute blood around relatively long segments of the proximal coronary artery, or percutaneous coronary intervention (PCI), a technique that uses catheter-borne mechanical devices to open a (usually) short area of stenosis from within the coronary artery, nowadays usually including implantation of a coronary stent. Both strategies have strengths and weaknesses, and it is not always clear which one would be optimal for a given patient. Studies comparing the two may be limited either by a lack of long-term follow-up, or by the "shifting sand" phenomenon, when long-term follow-up has been achieved, but by the time the study is completed, treatments in both arms have evolved to the point where the trial is not felt to be entirely relevant to contemporary practice.

Revascularization may be chosen to alleviate symptoms or to prolong life expectancy. Among patients with stable angina, the decision to proceed with revascularization is usually made in one of three situations: patients with anatomy for which revascularization has a proven survival benefit, those with activity-limiting symptoms despite maximum medical therapy, and active patients who want PCI for improved quality of life compared with medical therapy.

The Coronary Artery Surgery Study (CASS) compared surgery to angioplasty by coronary anatomy. On the basis of that trial, there is little doubt that surgery is preferred over medical treatment for patients with significant (>50%) left main stenosis, with an increased in median survival from 6.6 to 13.3 years (CASS Principal Investigators, 1983). Patients with diffuse triple-vessel disease and impaired LV function (ejection fraction <50%) also appear to benefit from CABG surgery. Left main equivalent disease, defined as proximal LAD and left circumflex disease (>70%), appears to behave similarly. Patients with proximal LAD disease and significant disease in one other vessel also appear to derive a mortality benefit from CABG (European Coronary Surgery Study Group, 1980).

In patients without surgical anatomy, the indication for revascularization is relief of symptoms. Stent-assisted PCI is generally preferred in patients with one- or two-vessel disease. The randomized trials comparing percutaneous transluminal coronary angioplasty and CABG for patients with multivessel coronary disease demonstrate equivalent short- and intermediate-term outcomes for coronary morbidity and mortality, with the important exception of diabetics requiring drug therapy. In the Bypass Angioplasty Revascularization Intervention (BARI) trial, patients with diabetes had improved survival with CABG (81 versus 66%) when surgery included a left internal mammary graft (BARI Investigators, 1996).

In other situations, factors favoring surgery include high-risk anatomy and unfavorable lesion morphology. Factors favoring PCI include significant co-morbidities, particular pulmonary, and other factors that may shorten life expectancy. Younger patients who may be expected to need multiple revascularization procedures over their life span owing to disease progression may be selected for initial percutaneous revascularization. In general, patients assigned to PCI have a shorter hospital stay and convalescence and an increased incidence of angina and of the need for subsequent revascularization

The impact of drug-eluting stents, which have a very low incidence of restenosis, is not entirely certain, but has the potential to shift the balance toward PCI. On the other hand, surgical techniques, particularly with respect to the use of arterial conduits and off-pump bypass procedures, are evolving as well. Regardless of revascularization technique, adjunctive risk-factor reduction remains crucial.

REFERENCES

1. Braunwald E. Control of myocardial oxygen consumption. Physiologic and clinical considerations. Am J Cardiol 27:416–432, 1971.
2. Braunwald E, Domanski MJ, Fowler SE, et al. Angiotensin-converting-enzyme inhibition in stable coronary artery disease. N Engl J Med 351:2058–2068, 2004.
3. Bypass Angioplasty Revascularization Investigation (BARI) Investigators. Comparison of coronary bypass surgery with angioplasty in patients with multivessel disease. N Engl J Med 335:217–225, 1996.
4. Cannon CP, Braunwald E, McCabe CH, et al. Intensive versus moderate lipid lowering with statins after acute coronary syndromes. N Engl J Med 350:1495–1504, 2004.
5. CASS Principal Investigators. Coronary artery surgery study (CASS): a randomized trial of coronary artery bypass surgery. Survival data. Circulation 68:939–950, 1983.
6. Chobanian AV, Bakris GL, Black HR, et al. Seventh report of the Joint National Committee on Prevention, Detection, Evaluation, and Treatment of High Blood Pressure. Hypertension 42:1206–1252, 2003.
7. Cohn PF, Gorlin R. Physiologic and clinical actions of nitroglycerin. Med Clin North Am 58:407–415, 1974.

8. Craven L. Experience with aspirin (acetysalicylic acid) in the non-specific prophylaxis of coronary thrombosis. Miss Vlly Med J 75:38–44, 1953.

9. DeWood MA, Stifter WF, Simpson CS, et al. Coronary arteriographic findings soon after non-Q-wave myocardial infarction. N Engl J Med 315:417–423, 1986.

10. Diabetes Control and Complications Trial Research Group. The effect of intensive treatment of diabetes on the development and progression of long-term complications in insulin-dependent diabetes mellitus. N Engl J Med 329:977–986, 1993.

11. European Coronary Surgery Study Group. Prospective randomised study of coronary artery bypass surgery in stable angina pectoris. Lancet 2:491–495, 1980.

12. Fox KM. Efficacy of perindopril in reduction of cardiovascular events among patients with stable coronary artery disease: randomised, double-blind, placebo-controlled, multicentre trial (the EUROPA study). Lancet 362:782–788, 2003.

13. Frick MH, Elo O, Haapa K, et al. Helsinki heart study: primary-prevention trial with gemfibrozil in middle-aged men with dyslipidemia. Safety of treatment, changes in risk factors, and incidence of coronary heart disease. N Engl J Med 317:1237–1245, 1987.

14. Frishman WH. Multifactorial actions of beta-adrenergic blocking drugs in ischemic heart disease: current concepts. Circulation 67:I11–18, 1983.

15. Gibbons RJ, Abrams J, Chatterjee K, et al. ACC/AHA 2002 guideline update for the management of patients with chronic stable angina—summary article: a report of the American College of Cardiology/American Heart Association Task Force on Practice Guidelines (Committee on the Management of Patients With Chronic Stable Angina). Circulation 107:149–158, 2003.

16. Grundy SM, Cleeman JI, Merz CN, et al. Implications of recent clinical trials for the National Cholesterol Education Program Adult Treatment Panel III guidelines. Circulation 110:227–239, 2004.

17. Hambrecht R, Walther C, Mobius-Winkler S, et al. Percutaneous coronary angioplasty compared with exercise training in patients with stable coronary artery disease: a randomized trial. Circulation 109:1371–1378, 2004.

18. Krauss RM, Eckel RH, Howard B, et al. AHA Dietary Guidelines: revision 2000: A statement for healthcare professionals from the Nutrition Committee of the American Heart Association. Circulation 102:2284–2299, 2000.

19. Lewis HD, Jr., Davis JW, Archibald DG, et al. Protective effects of aspirin against acute myocardial infarction and death in men with unstable angina. Results of a Veterans Administration cooperative study. N Engl J Med 309: 396–403, 1983.

20. Lipid Research Clinics Program. The lipid research clinics coronary primary prevention trial results. II. The relationship of reduction in incidence of coronary heart disease to cholesterol lowering. JAMA 251:365–374, 1984.

21. Long-Term Intervention with Pravastatin in Ischaemic Disease (LIPID) Study Group. Prevention of cardiovascular events and death with pravastatin in patients

with coronary heart disease and a broad range of initial cholesterol levels. N Engl J Med 339:1349–1357, 1998.

22. Neal B, MacMahon S, Chapman N. Effects of ACE inhibitors, calcium antagonists, and other blood-pressure-lowering drugs: results of prospectively designed overviews of randomised trials. Blood Pressure Lowering Treatment Trialists' Collaboration. Lancet 356:1955–1964, 2000.

23. Nissen SE, Tuzcu EM, Schoenhagen P, et al. Effect of intensive compared with moderate lipid-lowering therapy on progression of coronary atherosclerosis: a randomized controlled trial. JAMA 291:1071–1080, 2004.

24. Ockene IS, Miller NH. Cigarette smoking, cardiovascular disease, and stroke: a statement for healthcare professionals from the American Heart Association. American Heart Association Task Force on Risk Reduction. Circulation 96:3243–3247, 1997.

25. Oliva PB, Potts DE, Pluss RG. Coronary arterial spasm in Prinzmetal angina. Documentation by coronary arteriography. N Engl J Med 288:745–751,1973.

26. Platelet Receptor Inhibition in Ischemic Syndrome Management in Patients Limited by Unstable Signs and Symptoms (PRISM-PLUS) Study Investigators. Inhibition of the platelet glycoprotein IIb/IIIa receptor with tirofiban in unstable angina and non-Q-wave myocardial infarction. N Engl J Med 338:1488–1497, 1998.

27. Ridker PM, Cushman M, Stampfer MJ, Tracy RP, Hennekens CH. Inflammation, aspirin, and the risk of cardiovascular disease in apparently healthy men. N Engl J Med 336:973–979, 1997.

28. Sacks FM, Pfeffer MA, Moye LA, et al. The effect of pravastatin on coronary events after myocardial infarction in patients with average cholesterol levels. N Engl J Med 335:1001–1009, 1996.

29. Scandinavian Simvastatin Survival Study Group. Randomised trial of cholesterol lowering in 4444 patients with coronary heart disease: the Scandinavian Simvastatin Survival Study (4S). Lancet 344:1383–1389, 1994.

30. Stason WB, Schmid CH, Niedzwiecki D, et al. Safety of nifedipine in angina pectoris: a meta-analysis. Hypertension 33:24–31, 1999.

31. Steering Committee of the Physicians' Health Study Research Group. Final report on the aspirin component of the ongoing physicians' health study. N Engl J Med 321:129–135, 1989.

32. Theroux P, Ouimet H, McCans J, et al. Aspirin, heparin, or both to treat acute unstable angina. N Engl J Med 319:1105–1111, 1988.

33. Thompson PD, Buchner D, Pina IL, et al. Exercise and physical activity in the prevention and treatment of atherosclerotic cardiovascular disease: a statement from the Council on Clinical Cardiology (Subcommittee on Exercise, Rehabilitation, and Prevention) and the Council on Nutrition, Physical Activity, and Metabolism (Subcommittee on Physical Activity). Circulation 107:3109–3116, 2003.

34. UK Prospective Diabetes Study (UKPDS) Group. Intensive blood-glucose control with sulphonylureas or insulin compared with conventional treatment and risk of complications in patients with type 2 diabetes. Lancet 352:837–853, 1998.

35. Voskuil JH, Cramer MJ, Breumelhof R, Timmer R, Smout AJ. Prevalence of esophageal disorders in patients with chest pain newly referred to the cardiologist. Chest 109:1210–1214, 1996.

36. Yusuf S, Sleight P, Pogue J, et al., and The Heart Outcomes Prevention Evaluation Study Investigators. Effects of an angiotensin-converting-enzyme inhibitor, ramipril, on cardiovascular events in high-risk patients. N Engl J Med 342:145–153, 2000.

9   Valvular Diseases

AORTIC STENOSIS
Etiology and Pathophysiology

Aortic stenosis (AS) occurs when there is obstruction of blood flow across the aortic valve. AS can result from a congenitally abnormal valve, rheumatic fever, or degenerative/calcific disease. The incidence of these various etiologies differs with age at presentation. In children, AS results from a congenital abnormality, either supravalvular or subvalvular lesions, or occasionally, a unicuspid valve in which two of the three commissures are fused, resulting in obstruction and symptoms in infancy. Bicuspid aortic valve is the most common congenital heart defect, occurring in 2% of the population with a male predominance and familial clustering (Otto et al., 1994). A bicuspid aortic valve tends to thicken and calcify, with symptoms of AS presenting in the third to fifth decades of life (Fenoglio et al., 1977). In AS resulting from rheumatic heart disease, there is commissural fusion, with symptoms usually developing in the fifth to sixth decade. Degenerative AS is calcific disease of trileaflet aortic valves, leading to restricted leaflet mobility. The histological features of calcific AS are similar to those seen in atherosclerosis (Otto et al., 1999). The prevalence of AS increases with age, affecting 1.3% of people aged 65 to 74, and 4% of people above the age of 85. Aortic sclerosis is the thickening of the aortic valve without restriction of motion. The prevalence of aortic sclerosis also increases with age, affecting with 20% of people aged 65 to 74, and 48% above age 85 (Lindroos et al., 1993; Stewart et al., 1997). Risk factors for developing aortic sclerosis include age, smoking, low-density lipoprotein, diabetes, hypertension, male sex, and lipoprotein A level (Stewart et al., 1997). An echocardiographic study showed that 16% of patients with aortic sclerosis develop AS

From: *Current Clinical Practice: Cardiology in Family Practice:*
A Practical Guide
By: S. M. Hollenberg and T. Walker © Humana Press Inc., Totowa, NJ

(Cosmi et al., 2002). Aortic sclerosis by itself carries an increased risk of cardiovascular morbidity and mortality (Otto et al., 1999).

As obstruction to left ventricular (LV) outflow increases, a greater developed systolic pressure is required, increasing wall stress (pressure × radius/wall thickness by the Laplace law). LV hypertrophy ensues as a compensatory mechanism to normalize wall stress. This hypertrophy leads to decreased compliance of the left ventricle. Increased wall stress and LV mass increase oxygen demand, and this, in combination with decreased aortic pressure resulting from the pressure gradient across the valve, can set up a milieu for subendocardial ischemia.

Clinical Features

Patients with AS remain relatively asymptomatic, even as obstruction progresses, because the hypertrophied heart can generate the intraventricular pressures to maintain a normal stroke volume. The first symptoms usually occur because of the diastolic dysfunction, but clinical manifestations of decreases in cardiac output and coronary blood flow eventually ensue. When this occurs patients may experience dyspnea, angina and exertional syncope. The average survival is less than 2 to 3 years after the onset of symptoms.

The classic physical findings are a delayed and diminished carotid upstroke ("pulsus parvus et tardus") and a harsh systolic ejection murmur. This murmur is heard best at the heart base and often radiates to the carotids. The loudness of the murmur is not a reliable index of the severity of stenosis because the murmur gets softer as patients decompensate and cardiac output diminishes. The murmur does peak later in systole as the severity of the AS increases. LV hypertrophy is manifest as a sustained and laterally displaced apical impulse.

If the valve is still mobile, a systolic ejection click may be audible. The second heart sound may be soft as a result of decreased cuspal excursion, and there may be paradoxical splitting of S2 owing to prolongation of the LV ejection time. An S4 may result from decreased LV compliance, and heart failure may produce an S3 gallop.

Electrocardiogram (ECG) most often shows LV hypertrophy with strain pattern. Extensive calcifications can result in intraventricular conduction delay. Chest radiography may show aortic calcifications and rounding of the LV apex in addition to cardiomegaly.

Echocardiography with Doppler is used to assess LV size and function, valvular morphology, to measure transvalvular pressure gradients, and to calculate valvular area. Measurement of the gradient can be a trap because the gradient goes down when cardiac output falls; use of area to assess the severity of valvular stenosis is usually preferable. The normal aortic valve area is 3–4 cm². Severity is graded by valve area: mild, 1.2–2.0 cm², moderate, 1.0–1.2 cm², severe, 0.8–1.0 cm², critical less than 0.75 cm². Patients with mild AS should get an echocardiogram every 5 years, moderate AS every 2 years, and severe AS annually (Bonow et al., 1998). Echocardiography should also be performed whenever there is a clinical change in the patient. Cardiac catheterization is only rarely needed to confirm the severity of the AS, but is usually indicated to assess the coronary arteries in preparation for aortic valve replacement. Exercise testing is not recommended unless the patient is asymptomatic, and must be performed with careful supervision.

Treatment

There is no effective medical therapy to relieve obstruction in patients with AS, and treatment is recommended only for asymptomatic patients with systemic hypertension. There are some suggestions that therapy with statins may reduce progression (Bellamy et al., 2002; Rosenhek et al., 2004), but long-term outcome studies have not yet been completed. Vasodilators and diuretics should be used with extreme caution in these patients because hypotension can lead to ischemia, decreasing cardiac output and worsening hypotension, with the potential for a vicious cycle. All patients with AS should receive bacterial endocarditis prophylaxis, according to the American College of Cardiology/American Heart Association (ACC/AHA) guidelines (Bonow et al., 1998). Asymptomatic patients should be counseled regarding physical activity. The ACC/AHA guidelines recommend the following: (a) asymptomatic patients with mild AS can participate in competitive sports, (b) asymptomatic patients with moderate AS should avoid competitive sports, and (b) asymptomatic patients with severe AS should limit their activity (Bonow et al., 1998).

The ACC/AHA recommends that all symptomatic patients be considered for aortic valve replacement, and this is a class I indication (Bonow et al., 1998). Patients with severe AS who are asymptomatic should also be considered for aortic valve replacement if they have LV systolic dysfunction, hypotension during exercise, ventricular tachycardia, excessive LV hypertrophy, or a valve area less than 0.6 cm² (Bonow et al., 1998). If a mechanical prosthesis is inserted, patients will be committed to lifelong anticoagulation.

AORTIC REGURGITATION
Etiology and Pathophysiology

Aortic regurgitation (AR) is caused by non-coaptation of the aortic leaflets. It can from diseases of the aortic leaflets or aortic root, and its onset may be acute or chronic.

Acute AR may result from endocarditis, trauma, dissection of the aortic root, rupture of the sinus of Valsalva or of a myxomatous valve cusp, and acute dysfunction of a prosthetic or tissue valve.

In acute AR, the incompetent aortic valve causes acute volume overload and consequent diastolic pressure overload of the left ventricle. The left ventricle cannot adapt for this volume overload and therefore cannot maintain an adequate effective stroke volume and cardiac output. Compensatory tachycardia results, in an attempt to try to maintain effective cardiac output. The LV diastolic pressure rise increases left atrial (LA) and pulmonary arterial pressure, leading to pulmonary edema and cardiogenic shock.

Chronic AR is the result of a progressive deterioration of the aortic leaflets or root. Causes range from a bicuspid valve, rheumatic heart disease, endocarditis, Marfan's syndrome, connective tissue diseases, syphilis, and hypertension.

Chronic AR is generally well tolerated because the left ventricle has time to dilate in response to the chronic volume overload produced by the regurgitant volume into the left ventricle. This compensatory response increases forward stroke volume and maintains effective cardiac output. The increased LV volume increases wall stress, with compensatory eccentric LV hypertrophy. Over time, the left ventricle dilates and hypertrophies. When compensation fails, LV diastolic pressure increases and symptoms may ensue.

Clinical Features

Early in chronic AR, patients are relatively asymptomatic, yet there may be vague complaints of fatigue, awareness of the heart beating, and palpitations. The usual presenting symptom is dyspnea.

Classic auscultatory signs of chronic AR include a soft S2 in addition to the classic blowing decrescendo diastolic murmur, which is best heard with the patient leaning forward during end expiration. A systolic flow murmur is frequently audible as well. P2 may be loud if the patient has developed pulmonary hypertension. Rapid LV filling may produce a third heart sound. Severe AR may cause mitral valve preclosure and an apical diastolic murmur of relative MS across a structurally normal valve (Austin-Flint murmur).

The classic peripheral signs of severe chronic AR include a wide pulse pressure (Corrigan's pulse), systolic head bobbing (Demusset sign), systolic pulsations of the uvula (Mueller's sign), pistol shot pulses (Traube sign), capillary pulsations (Quicke's pulses), to-and-fro femoral bruits (Duroziez's sign), and Hills sign (lower extremity blood pressure [BP] greater than upper extremity BP).

In acute AR, many of the characteristic physical findings of chronic AR are modified or absent. Pulse pressure may not be increased because systolic pressure is reduced and the aortic diastolic pressure equilibrates with the elevated LV diastolic pressure, but tachycardia is invariably present. Owing to equilibration between the aortic and ventricular diastolic pressure, the diastolic murmur may be short and soft or even inaudible. Mitral valve preclosure may produce a soft S1.

In chronic AR, chest radiography shows cardiomegaly, with or without signs of pulmonary vascular congestion. The aortic root may be dilated. In acute AR, cardiomegaly may be absent on chest x-ray, but pulmonary edema is usual. Similarly, the ECG in chronic AR will show LV hypertrophy, often with nonspecific ST-T changes of LV strain, and LA enlargement. In acute AR, only sinus tachycardia and nonspecific ST changes may be present.

Echocardiography is the most useful technique for the diagnosis of acute and chronic AR. Two-dimensional echocardiography can be used to assess chambers sizes and LV function, and also quantifies aortic root size. It can also help to define the etiology. If aortic dissection or endocarditis with aortic ring abscess is suspected, transesophageal echocardiography is recommended. Doppler echocardiography can reliably define the severity of the AR. LV dimensions and systolic performance are important criteria used in evaluation for surgical intervention (Bonow et al., 1998). Cardiac catheterization can be used to confirm the severity of the regurgitation, but is generally most useful to look for concomitant coronary artery disease (CAD).

Treatment

Acute AR is a medical emergency that presents with pulmonary edema and decreased cardiac output. As previously noted, many of the classic signs of chronic AR are attenuated or absent. Patients are stabilized with diuretics, parenteral nitrates to reduce preload, and afterload reducers such as sodium nitroprusside or angiotensin-converting enzyme (ACE) inhibitors if BP permits (Khan & Gray, 1991). Inotropic agents such a dopamine or dobutamine may be necessary to support cardiac output and temporarily lower LV end-diastolic pressure until surgical intervention can be performed. Intra-aortic balloon counterpulsation is contraindicated in patients with AR. Bradycardia increases the regurgitant fraction and should be avoided; in fact, pacing may be helpful in some cases. Patients with dissection involving the ascending aorta or endocarditis with AR and pulmonary edema require emergent surgery.

In chronic severe AR, chronic therapy with vasodilators, such as ACE inhibitors, nifedipine, or hydralazine can reduce LV end-diastolic volume and mass, and maintain ejection fraction (EF; Bonow et al., 1998; Lin et al., 1994; Scognamiglio et al., 1990). Indications for vasodilating agents for chronic severe AR include (a) symptomatic patients who are poor surgical candidates with severe AR and LV dysfunction, (b) patients with severe heart failure symptoms prior to surgical intervention, and (c) asymptomatic patients with volume overloaded left ventricles but normal LV function (Bonow et al., 1998). The doses should be titirated to the maximum tolerated dose. Vasodilator therapy with nifedipine has been shown to delay the need for aortic valve replacement in patients with asymptomatic severe AR (Scognamiglio et al., 1994).

In asymptomatic patients with mild AR and normal LV function, vasodilating agents are not recommended unless systemic hypertension is present. These patients should be followed with annual history and physical examination, with serial echocardiography every 2–3 years (Bonow et al., 1998). In symptomatic patients with moderate AR, vasodilators are probably useful to delay disease progression, but no outcome data are available. Physical examination and echocardiography are recommended annually (Bonow et al., 1998). Asymptomatic patients with severe AR and normal LV function should be clinically assessed every 6 months with an ECG every 6–12 months. A repeat echo should be performed on any patient with new symptoms (Bonow et al., 1998). Patients should be advised to avoid isometric exercises. All patients with AR are advised to avoid isometric exercise, and all require bacterial endocarditis prophylaxis (Bonow et al., 1998).

The ACC/AHA recommendations for surgery are based on the onset of symptoms or LV dysfunction or dilatation. Aortic valve replacement is recommended for patients with severe AR in the following situations: (a) symptomatic patients with normal LV function or LV dysfunction, (b) asymptomatic patients with measurable LV dysfunction (EF <55%), and (c) asymptomatic patients with an end-systolic dimension greater than 50 mm or an end-diastolic diameter greater than 70 mm (Bonow et al., 1998).

MITRAL STENOSIS

Etiology and Pathophysiology

Mitral stenosis (MS) is a narrowing of the mitral valve, which impedes flow from the left atrium to the left ventricle during diastole. The most common cause of MS is rheumatic fever, although a history of rheumatic fever may not be elicited. There is a latency period of about 10 to 20 years before the patient develops symptoms of MS. Less common etiologies include atrial myxoma, carcinoid, congenital MS, systemic lupus, rheumatoid arthritis, and mucopolysacharroidosis.

The normal mitral valve area is 4–6 cm². A valve area greater than 2 cm² is considered mildly stenotic, between 1 and 2 cm² is moderate, and less than 1 cm² is severe MS. As the valve area narrows, the LA pressure rises to maintain LV filling and cardiac output. The increase in LA pressure results in increased pressure in the pulmonary vasculature. Over time, this can lead to pulmonary edema, pulmonary hypertension, and right-sided heart failure. Long-standing severe pulmonary hypertension may lead to pulmonary fibrosis and may be irreversible.

The left ventricle is generally protected in pure MS. If the valve becomes sufficiently stenotic, LV filling and end-diastolic volume can diminish, leading to a decrease in stroke volume and cardiac output.

Clinical Features

Symptoms of MS generally occur when the valve area is less than 2.5 cm^2 (Gorlin & Gorlin, 1951). The initial symptom in MS is usually exertional dyspnea. Increased heart rate with exercise decreases diastolic filling time and consequently increases LA and pulmonary vascular pressure. Other symptoms of MS include hemoptysis, orthopnea, paroxysmal nocturnal dyspnea, fatigue, palpitations, and thromboembolic events. In fact, thromboembolism as a result of atrial fibrillation may be the first manifestation of MS.

On physical examination, the first heart sound is loud because of increased LA pressure prior to mitral valve closure. A mid-diastolic opening snap may be heard as the LV pressure falls below the LA pressure and the mitral valve opens vigorously. As the severity of the MS increases and the LA pressure rises, the opening snap comes closer to S2. The classic murmur of MS is a low pitched mid-diastolic rumble best heard at the apex with the patient lying in the left lateral decubitus position. Other signs of severe MS are referable to pulmonary hypertension, and include a loud P2, jugular venous distension with a prominent a wave, and a right ventricular heave.

The classic ECG findings of MS are a broad notched P wave indicative of LA enlargement and hypertrophy. Atrial fibrillation may also be present. As the patient develops pulmonary hypertension and right ventricular hypertrophy, the QRS axis shifts to the right with tall R waves in V_1 and V_2. Chest radiography in MS shows straightening of the left heart border, pulmonary venous congestion, and dilated pulmonary arteries. As the left atrium enlarges it may displace the esophagus posteriorly.

Echocardiography is the definitive and essential diagnostic test to define valve anatomy and delineate the severity of the MS. Doppler echocardiography can measure the transmitral gradient, mitral valve area, and the pulmonary artery pressure, which provides important information for evaluation of an asymptomatic patient. Morphological evaluation of the mitral valve and subvalvular apparatus, with application of a scoring system encompassing leaflet thickening, subvalvular deformity, calcification, and leaflet mobility is used to assess suitability for valvuloplasty (Wilkins et al., 1988).

Therapy

Because the left ventricle is protected, MS can be well tolerated for a long time. When symptoms occur, medical therapy can provide very effective relief. Diuretics are beneficial for symptoms of pulmonary vascular congestion. Because exertional dyspnea usually results from increased heart rate, β-blockade or calcium channel blockers (CCBs) with negative chronotropic actions prevent excessive tachycardia and provide symptomatic relief by increasing diastolic filling time. Atrial fibrillation with loss of atrial kick is poorly tolerated in MS. Cardioversion should be considered, but if unsuccessful, digoxin, β-blockers, or CCBs, are used to control ventricular rate.

Anticoagulation, unless contraindicated, should be given to patients with MS and atrial fibrillation or to patients with a prior embolic event (Bonow et al., 1998). Because increased LA size predisposes to atrial fibrillation, which may not always be symptomatic, anticoagulation is also recommended (class II indication) for patients with MS and LA diameter greater than 5.5 cm (Salem et al., 2004). The target international normalized ratio (INR) should be 2.5, with a range from 2 to 3. If a patient has an embolic event while on anticoagulation, aspirin (75–100 mg/day) is usually added, and the target INR is increased to 3.0 (range 2.5–3.5). If the patient cannot tolerate aspirin, clopidogrel 75 mg per day should be substituted (Salem et al., 2004).

Asymptomatic patients with mild MS need to be followed annually with a history, physical exam, ECG, and chest x-ray. Echocardiography is recommended at the initial presentation and thereafter if there is a change in clinical status. If patients have palpitations, then ambulatory ECG monitoring is recommended to rule out intermittent atrial fibrillation. Patients with severe MS should be followed with a clinical exam every 6 months and echocardiography every 12 months. Patients with severe MS can be asymptomatic as a result of adjustments in lifestyle and therefore these patients should be evaluated by echocardiography to measure pulmonary arterial pressures. Bacterial endocarditis and rheumatic fever prophylaxis is required for all patients with MS.

Guidelines for interventional therapy, surgical repair, or valve replacement have been promulgated by the ACC/AHA (Bonow et al., 1998). Valvotomy is recommended for asymptomatic patients with moderate or severe MS with pulmonary artery pressure greater than 50 mmHg or poor exercise tolerance, symptomatic patients with moderate to severe MS, or symptomatic patients with mild MS and increased pulmonary artery pressure. Relative contraindications to valvotomy are LA thrombus and moderate to severe mitral regurgitation (Bonow et al., 1998). Surgical repair is recommended for symptomatic patients with moderate to severe MS with favorable valve morphology for repair if balloon valvotomy is not available, and symptomatic moderate to severe MS if LA thrombus is present (Bonow et al., 1998). Mitral valve replacement is recommended for symptomatic patients with moderate to severe MS and valve morphology unfavorable for valvotomy, and for patients with severe MS and mild symptoms but severe pulmonary hypertension and unfavorable valve morphology (Bonow et al., 1998).

MITRAL REGURGITATION

Etiology and Pathophysiology

Mitral regurgitation (MR) can be acute or chronic; both the presentations and etiologies differ. Acute MR may result from chordal rupture in patients with myxomatous valves, acute infective endocarditis, and blunt or perforating chest trauma resulting in leaflet tear or chordal rupture, as well as papillary muscle rupture or dysfunction in the setting of inferior infarction. Chronic MR occurs in the setting of mitral valve prolapse, rheumatic heart disease, infectious endocarditis, collagen vascular disease, dilated cardiomyopathy, and mitral annular calcification.

In acute MR, the sudden increase in regurgitant blood volume from the left ventricle increases LA pressure and causes acute pulmonary hypertension. LV ejection into the lower pressure left atrium impairs forward flow, which can lead to a decrease in cardiac output and cardiogenic shock.

In chronic MR, compensatory dilation of the left atrium increases its compliance and decreases LA pressure. The left ventricle compensates for its volume overload by eccentric hypertrophy and dilation, helping to maintain cardiac output. Eventually, the increased volume can increase LV wall stress and impair ventricular performance. It is important to recognize that ejection fraction is not a reliable measure of ventricular performance in MR; ejection fraction can be maintained even in the face of impaired contractility because the LV is ejecting into the LA.

Clinical Features

Patients with acute MR presents dramatically with the sudden onset of pulmonary edema, hypotension, and cardiogenic shock. The murmur of acute MR may be limited to early systole because of rapid equalization of pressures in the left atrium and left ventricle. More importantly, the murmur may be soft or inaudible, especially when cardiac output is low.

Chronic MR, on the other hand, is generally well tolerated, and patients may remain asymptomatic for years. Over time, as the left ventricle enlarges, patients may present with of heart failure symptoms of heart failure, such as fatigue, dyspnea, orthopnea, and edema. Increased pulmonary pressures may result in hemoptysis. LA enlargement sometimes causes impingement on the left recurrent laryngeal nerve, leading to hoarseness.

On physical examination the apical impulse is hyperkinetic and displaced laterally in chronic MR. A holosystolic apical murmur that usually radiates to the axilla can be auscultated, and sometimes a systolic thrill is palpable; an S3 is frequently present. In patients with mitral valve prolapse, a mid-systolic click may be heard. With the development of pulmonary hypertension, jugular venous pressure is elevated and the pulmonary component of the second heart sound is loud. A right ventricle heave may be present as well.

The ECG usually reflects the anatomical changes in the heart with evidence of LV hypertrophy, LA enlargement, and possibly atrial fibrillation. The chest radiograph will show cardiomegaly, with or without pulmonary congestion. The pulmonary arteries may be dilated. In acute MR, pulmonary edema is evident.

Echocardiography is essential and usually definitive. Echocardiography is used to define mitral valve morphology, identify chordal and papillary muscle rupture, measure the degree of annular dilatation and LA size. Doppler echocardiography can reliably define the severity of the MR, and may be used to estimate pulmonary artery pressures as well. LV function and end-systolic dimensions are needed to assess the timing of potential operative repair. Transesophageal echocardiography can be helpful when transthoracic images are suboptimal. Cardiac catheterization with ventriculography can confirm the degree of MR, but is generally used to assess the degree of CAD prior to surgical repair or in suspected ischemic papillary muscle rupture.

Therapy

Management of acute severe MR entails stabilization of the patient with intravenous afterload reduction (nitroprusside or enalaprilat) and intra-aortic balloon counterpulsation, but these are temporizing measures. Inotropic or vasopressor therapy may also be needed to support cardiac output and BP. Nitrates may be incorporated if ischemia is causing or contributing to acute MR. Definitive therapy, however, is surgical valve repair or replacement, which should be undertaken as soon as possible because clinical deterioration can be sudden.

Asymptomatic patients with mild MR without pulmonary hypertension, LV dysfunction or dilatation should be followed annually (Bonow et al., 1998). Echocardiography should be done initially and repeated if there is a change in clinical status. Patients with moderate MR should have an annual exam and echocardiography (Bonow et al., 1998). Asymptomatic patients with severe MR should be followed every 6–12 months with a clinical exam and echocardiography (Bonow et al., 1998).

Vasodilating drugs are not indicated for asymptomatic patients with MR, unless there is systemic hypertension. Patients with symptomatic MR, or those with LV dysfunction, however, do benefit from vasodilators (Greenberg et al., 1982). In chronic mild to moderate MR, afterload reduction with ACE inhibitors or nifedipine makes sense to prevent LV dilatation, but has not been shown to improve mortality. Some experts advocate β-blockade. In chronic severe MR, ACE inhibitors are usually used, although there is no definitive evidence for their benefit. Patients with MR often have other indications for ACE inhibitors and β-blockers, such as cardiomyopathy. Diuretics and digoxin are used as needed for heart failure. Bacterial endocarditis prophylaxis is required for all patients with MR.

Surgery is recommended for all symptomatic patients with severe MR regardless of the LV function (Bonow et al., 1998). Asymptomatic patients with severe MR and LV end-systolic dimension greater than 45 mm or EF less than 55–60% are also candidates for surgical intervention, as are those with normal LV function and pulmonary hypertension and/or atrial fibrillation (Bonow et al., 1998). Asymptomatic patients with normal LV function and normal pulmonary pressures can be followed clinically every 6 months (Bonow et al., 1998).

Mitral valve repair is the procedure of choice when the valve morphology is amenable to repair. Most clinicians lower their threshold for operative intervention when valve repair is felt to be feasible. Mitral valve repair leads to better LV performance and does not require lifelong anticoagulation (Enriquez-Sarano et al., 1995). More calcified valves may need replacement, but chordal sparing and reattachment improves ventricular performance. Some patients with very dilated left ventricles and MR may benefit from mitral annuloplasty.

REFERENCES

1. Bellamy MF, Pellikka PA, Klarich KW, Tajik AJ, Enriquez-Sarano M. Association of cholesterol levels, hydroxymethylglutaryl coenzyme-A reductase inhibitor treatment, and progression of aortic stenosis in the community. J Am Coll Cardiol 40:1723–1730, 2002.
2. Bonow RO, Carabello B, de Leon AC, Jr., et al. Guidelines for the management of patients with valvular heart disease: executive summary. A report of the American College of Cardiology/American Heart Association Task Force on Practice Guidelines (Committee on Management of Patients with Valvular Heart Disease). Circulation 98:1949–1984, 1998.
3. Cosmi JE, Kort S, Tunick PA, et al. The risk of the development of aortic stenosis in patients with "benign" aortic valve thickening. Arch Intern Med 162:2345–2347, 2002.
4. Enriquez-Sarano M, Schaff HV, Orszulak TA, Tajik AJ, Bailey KR, Frye RL. Valve repair improves the outcome of surgery for mitral regurgitation. A multivariate analysis. Circulation 91:1022–1028, 1995.
5. Fenoglio JJ, Jr., McAllister HA, Jr., DeCastro CM, Davia JE, Cheitlin MD. Congenital bicuspid aortic valve after age 20. Am J Cardiol 39:164–169, 1977.
6. Gorlin R, Gorlin SG. Hydraulic formula for calculation of the area of stenotic mitral valve, other cardiac values and central circulatory shunts. Am Heart J 1951;41:1–29.
7. Greenberg BH, DeMots H, Murphy E, Rahimtoola SH. Arterial dilators in mitral regurgitation: effects on rest and exercise hemodynamics and long-term clinical follow-up. Circulation 65:181–187, 1982.

8. Khan SS, Gray RJ. Valvular emergencies. Cardiol Clin 9:689–709, 1991.

9. Lin M, Chiang HT, Lin SL, et al. Vasodilator therapy in chronic asymptomatic aortic regurgitation: enalapril versus hydralazine therapy. J Am Coll Cardiol 24:1046–1053, 1994.

10. Lindroos M, Kupari M, Heikkila J, Tilvis R. Prevalence of aortic valve abnormalities in the elderly: an echocardiographic study of a random population sample. J Am Coll Cardiol 21:1220–1225, 1993.

11. Otto CM, Kuusisto J, Reichenbach DD, Gown AM, O'Brien KD. Characterization of the early lesion of "degenerative" valvular aortic stenosis. Histological and immunohistochemical studies. Circulation 90:844–853, 1994.

12. Otto CM, Lind BK, Kitzman DW, Gersh BJ, Siscovick DS. Association of aortic-valve sclerosis with cardiovascular mortality and morbidity in the elderly. N Engl J Med 341:142–147, 1999.

13. Rosenhek R, Rader F, Loho N, et al. Statins but not angiotensin-converting enzyme inhibitors delay progression of aortic stenosis. Circulation 110:1291–1295, 2004.

14. Salem DN, Stein PD, Al-Ahmad A, et al. Antithrombotic therapy in valvular heart disease—native and prosthetic: the Seventh ACCP Conference on Antithrombotic and Thrombolytic Therapy. Chest 126:457S–482S, 2004.

15. Scognamiglio R, Fasoli G, Ponchia A, Dalla-Volta S. Long-term nifedipine unloading therapy in asymptomatic patients with chronic severe aortic regurgitation. J Am Coll Cardiol 16:424–429, 1990.

16. Scognamiglio R, Rahimtoola SH, Fasoli G, Nistri S, Dalla Volta S. Nifedipine in asymptomatic patients with severe aortic regurgitation and normal left ventricular function. N Engl J Med 331:689–694, 1994.

17. Stewart BF, Siscovick D, Lind BK, et al. Clinical factors associated with calcific aortic valve disease. Cardiovascular Health Study. J Am Coll Cardiol 29: 630–634, 1997.

18. Wilkins GT, Weyman AE, Abascal VM, Block PC, Palacios IF. Percutaneous balloon dilatation of the mitral valve: an analysis of echocardiographic variables related to outcome and the mechanism of dilatation. Br Heart J 60:299–308, 1988.

Index